Public Health
in
America

This is a volume in the Arno Press series

PUBLIC HEALTH IN AMERICA

Advisory Editor

Barbara Gutmann Rosenkrantz

Editorial Board

**Leona Baumgartner
James H. Cassedy
Arthur Jack Viseltear**

See last pages of this volume
for a complete list of titles.

HEALTH IN THE SOUTHERN UNITED STATES

ARNO PRESS

A New York Times Company

New York / 1977

Editorial Supervision: JOSEPH CELLINI

Reprint Edition 1977 by Arno Press Inc.

Copyright © 1977 by Arno Press Inc.

A Sketch of the Soil, Climate, Weather and Diseases of South Carolina was reprinted from a copy in the State Historical Society of Wisconsin Library. Organization, Activites, and Results was reprinted from a copy in the University of Illinois Library.

PUBLIC HEALTH IN AMERICA
ISBN for complete set: 0-405-09804-9
See last pages of this volume for titles.

Manufactured in the United States of America

Publisher's Note: This book has been reprinted from the best available copies. The maps have been reproduced in black and white for this edition.

Library of Congress Cataloging in Publication Data
Main entry under title:

Health in the Southern United States.

   (Public health in America)
   Reprint of pamphlets published 1790-1916.
   CONTENTS: Ramsay, D. A dissertation on the means of preserving health in Charleston and the adjacent low country.--Ramsay, D. A sketch of the soil, climate, weather, and diseases of South Carolina.--Nott, J. C. An examination into the health and longevity of the Southern sea ports of the United States, with reference to the subject of life insurance. [etc.]
   1. Medical geography--Southern States--Addresses, essays, lectures. 2. Public health--Southern States--Addresses, essays, lectures. I. Series.
RA807.S85H4   362.1'0975   76-40667
ISBN 0-405-09875-8

CONTENTS

Ramsay, David
A DISSERTATION ON THE MEANS OF PRESERVING HEALTH IN CHARLESTON AND THE ADJACENT LOW COUNTRY. Charleston, 1790

Ramsay, David
A SKETCH OF THE SOIL, CLIMATE, WEATHER, AND DISEASES OF SOUTH-CAROLINA. Charleston, 1796

Nott, J[osiah] C.
AN EXAMINATION INTO THE HEALTH AND LONGEVITY OF THE SOUTHERN SEA PORTS OF THE UNITED STATES WITH REFERENCE TO THE SUBJECT OF LIFE INSURANCE (Reprinted from the *Southern Journal of Medicine and Pharmacy,* Vol. II, No. 2), Charleston, March, 1847

Barton, E[dward] H.
REPORT TO THE LOUISIANA STATE MEDICAL SOCIETY ON THE METEOROLOGY, VITAL STATISTICS AND HYGIENE OF THE STATE OF LOUISIANA. New Orleans, 1851

Rose, Wickliffe
ORGANIZATION, ACTIVITIES, AND RESULTS UP TO DECEMBER 31, 1910 (Reprinted from the *Rockefeller Sanitary Commission for the Eradication of Hookworm*), Washington, D.C., 1910

Goldberger, Joseph
PELLAGRA: Causation and a Method of Prevention. A Summary of Some of the Recent Studies of the United States Public Health Service (Reprinted from *Journal of the American Medical Association,* Vol. LXVI, No. 7), Chicago, February 12, 1916

A DISSERTATION ON THE MEANS OF PRESERVING HEALTH IN CHARLESTON AND THE ADJACENT LOW COUNTRY

David Ramsey

A DISSERTATION

ON THE MEANS OF PRESERVING HEALTH IN CHARLESTON, AND THE ADJACENT LOW COUNTRY.

THE object of the medical profession is not only to heal diseases, but to prevent them. As it is my turn this evening to furnish a subject of conversation for the society, I shall, with great deference, submit to their consideration some practical observations on the means of preventing those diseases which are most common in Charleston and the vicinity. This I do the more readily as, having enjoyed almost uninterrupted health during a residence of sixteen years in this climate, I hope that I may be allowed to have some experimental knowledge of the subject.

The foundation of good health through life, should be laid in a proper treatment of infants. Their limbs should be unconfined, and frequently rubbed. Their food ought to be plain and simple. They should be kept constantly clean, and never suffered to remain wet for any length of time. Caps should be laid aside after the third or fourth month in winter, and much sooner in summer. Shoes and stockings may well be dispensed with through the whole period of infancy. Every prudent exertion should be early made for hardening the constitution against sudden changes of the atmosphere. To this end exercise should be freely and daily taken in the open air. When the weather turns suddenly cold, some additional cloathing may be proper; but it is often more for the interest of children, to habituate them to all the varieties of our weather, and even to expose them to occasional colds, than by an excess of care and tenderness to induce a delicacy of habit.

In nursing cradles are hurtful. They add much to the heat of the infants who are confined between their narrow sides. A hard matrass is much cooler and on many accounts preferable. The youths who are accustomed to sleep on the floor with bare blankets, will pass through life with more independence and with greater advantages than they who are accustomed to the relaxing indulgencies of soft beds.

On the propriety of using young children in this country to the cold bath, well informed physicians hold different opinions. In some habits it certainly does good by bracing the tender limbs and fortifying the body against sudden changes of the air, while in others the shock is too great. In general it may neverthless be safely affirmed that a great majority of our children would have a better chance for escaping the diseases of infancy, if they were from an early period of life habituated to the frequent use of the cold bath; and that very few cases occur in which the daily washing of them in cold water would not be of advantage.

Providence has kindly furnished us with an efficacious remedy for worms. Pink root is one of the best vermifuges in the world, and the seasonable administration of it to our children, would save them from what often proves a source of disease and death.

The

The months of April and May have been found by long experience to be unfriendly to children in Charleston. Parents should, therefore, make arrangements for keeping them out of the city during these two months. Country air is of singular utility not only for preventing but curing that vomiting and purging which attacks children on the approach of warm weather. Where a retreat to the country is not practicable, the next best preventive of this dangerous complaint is cold bathing.

The stomachs and intestines of infants should be well cleansed soon after they are born. That mothers should rest for several hours after their delivery is advisable. While they are recruited by repose after the sufferings of parturition, their offspring may be prepared for sucking with safety. This can only be done by thoroughly emptying their stomachs and intestines.

On this occasion give me leave to observe, that the writings of physicians who have practised in colder climates are not applicable to this country. They represent the first milk of mothers as sufficient to carry off the meconium of new born infants, but the contrary is known among us to every practitioner of physic. Milk either has not the same qualities, or does not produce the same effects in warm as in cold countries. In this climate it not only often fails in carrying off from new born infants those crudities the retention of which gives rise to many diseases, but instead thereof, by mingling with them, produces such disturbances in the alimentary canal, as frequently issue in immediate

diate death. Much of the mortality among children, especially on plantations, is owing to this cause. Overlaying, which is commonly said to be the occasion of their death, takes place much seldomer than has been supposed. The locked jaw of infants frequently arises from the irritation excited by the mixture of milk with meconium. If there is any one direction of primary consequence for preserving the health, and even the lives of infants, it is to empty their stomachs and bowels well before they are suffered to suck plentifully. A due attention to this matter would annually save many lives.

For the preservation of health and prevention of diseases among adults, much is to be avoided and much is to be done. In the former class several particulars are to be reckoned. The first I shall mention is lying long in bed in the morning.

The coolest period of the day is a little before sun rising. This naturally proves a temptation to spend those precious moments in sleep. If this is indulged, the body lies immersed in the air which has been fouled by its perspiration through the night, and in a situation which tends to relax it nearly as much as if it was in a vapor bath. By proper improvement of the morning, new life, vigor and spirits are imparted for bearing the noontide heat; but by continuing to sleep, or even to loll, this opportunity of recruiting is lost—the languor and debility which resulted from the preceding day continues to increase, till a change of season brings relief. The cool morning air acts like the cold bath in invigorating the body, and

has

has an advantage over it by being inhaled and applied to the vitals. In another view of this subject, it may be added, that a man who rises early will comparatively add seven years of the best time for study and business to a life of sixty-five. Tho' early rising is very wholsome, yet going abroad in the morning in the country, while the grass is covered with dew, frequently produces fevers. To obtain the good, unmixed with the evil, the most should be made of the cool morning air, but without wetting our feet with damp grass, or otherwise exposing ourselves to an undue absorption of that moisture which abounds for some time after the rising of the sun. As a further precaution against the chills of the morning, it would be prudent never to go abroad with an empty stomach. A glass of cold water, or slice of bread, or a draught of some bitter tea, taken immediately after rising, would be beneficial.

The above cautions of avoiding the morning dew may safely be dispensed with in many cases. A man who washes his feet in cold water every day will hardly ever suffer from walking abroad in the morning. Nor will he who changes his shoes, and wipes his feet soon after they are wet from dewy grass. It may farther be added, that if children were educated as they ought to be, when grown up they would have little to fear from wet feet or morning dews.

Immoderate drinking should be avoided in this climate. To add the stimulus of large quantities of spirituous liquors to the heat occasioned by a warm atmosphere, is to add fuel to fire. Every evil that naturally results from an excess of heat, is aggravated by a plentiful use of ardent spirits. These tend to inflame the blood, and concur with a warm sun in wearing out the vitals, hastening on a premature old age and an untimely death. How far it would be for the benefit of our country to exterminate the use of distilled spirits, I will not undertake to determine, but have no hesitation in pronouncing, that the sum of evil resulting from their abuse infinitely outweighs all the good that flows from them.

The habit of immoderate drinking when once begun, hurries on its unhappy votaries almost irresistibly. In the intervals of sobriety, they feel a faintness and oppression which is intolerably distressing. For this they find no relief but in a second intoxication. As the liquor loses its stimulus, the dose must be increased so as to procure an abatement of painful sensations. The remedy proves worse than the disease, and both continue to increase in a fatal progression from bad to worse, from ordinary grog to undiluted Jamaica spirits: even the latter becomes insufficient to warm the stomach, and instances sometimes occur where the hottest peppers have been added to the warmest spirits to take off their fancied coldness. To enumerate all the diseases which are brought on in this warm climate, by the abuse of ardent spirits, would far exceed the limits to which I must confine myself. Suffice it to observe, that among them is the destruction of the digestive powers, obstructions of the abdominal viscera, dropsies and madness. Nothing can more powerfully illustrate the pernicious

nicious effects of rum than the havoc it makes among the Indians, who, from a robust and hardy race, by the free use of that pernicious liquid, become mad, waste away and die. They who wish to preserve health, should summon up all their resolution to prevent the blandishments of company, or the seductions of appetite, from inducing them to deviate into the paths of intemperance; for, when once they have entered on that course, their return to the practice of that moderation and sobriety which health requires, is always difficult and often impossible.

Of the many forms in which ardent spirits are taken to the prejudice of health, none is more injurious than drams. Under the insidious shew of fortifying the body against foggy and damp weather, the practice of daily drinking drams has slain its thousands. It gives a temporary stimulus to the system, but this is soon followed with increased debility. It creates a false appetite, and tempts to the eating of more solid food than either nature craves or the stomach can digest. These are its first effects. In process of time consequences of an opposite nature are produced. A loss of appetite, at least for breakfast, is a common complaint among those who have long been in the habit of drinking drams. To the evils resulting from this source physicians have sometimes incautiously contributed by recommending the use of bitters. Though the bitters taken in substance, or in water, may be useful, the spirits in which they are mostly prepared insensibly lead to the practice of dram-drinking.

drinking. Huxham's tincture of the bark is, on these principles, the occasion of much mischief. It would be for the interest of patients that physicians should never prescribe the internal use of any medicines prepared in spirits, except such as are taken in small doses. They pay too dearly for being cured of fevers or bad appetites, who, by taking spirituous tinctures for that purpose, contract a fondness for drams. On this subject, it is worthy of remark, that health is often much injured by those who are at all hours of the day sipping spirituous liquors, though they are never intoxicated. It is a good general rule never to drink any thing stronger than water, except at our meals.

An intemperate use of animal food should be avoided in this climate, especially in summer. Excess in eating is as bad as excess in drinking. It excites a greater oppression, and requires a greater exertion of the digestive organs. The warmer the weather, the greater is the tendency to putrefaction. It cannot be expected, that meat which becomes tainted in a few hours in market, can be much longer otherwise when it is taken immoderately into the stomach. As often as an undue proportion of meat is taken at a meal, nature is not only oppressed, but a foundation is laid for putrid diseases. Perhaps in this view of the matter, a small proportion of salted meat, as being less disposed to putrefaction than fresh, would be more suitable aliment in summer than has generally been supposed.

Inactivity

Inactivity is another of the evils against which the votaries of health should fix their most determined opposition. Many of our summer diseases arise from suppressed perspiration. From whatever cause this proceeds, languor and lassitude are the immediate consequences. These unpleasant sensations ought to be instantly removed; but to accomplish that desirable object, recourse should immediately be had to such active exertions as are calculated to restore an equable and free perspiration. Our feelings on these occasions deceive us. They persuade us to indulge in rest, but a regard to health leads to activity. The sense of weariness, which arises from suppressed perspiration, is more easily overcome by resisting than yielding. The person who sits or lies down will find his lassitude to continue and increase; but he, who in opposition to his own feelings, makes a proper exertion of his active powers, will soon be relieved from it.

The effects of exercise in promoting digestion, and all the regular functions of animal life, are too well known to need illustration. Suffice it to observe, by way of applying the general observations to our local situation, that from the great moisture of our atmosphere, impediments to a free perspiration frequently occur. These should be counteracted by such constant, equable activity as, without heating the body, will keep all the secretions in their due order and proportion.

Among the evils resulting from indolence, a fondness for drinking ardent spirits is not the least,

least. Human nature is so constituted that it requires something to agitate it. Where the mind and body are both unemployed, the stimulus of strong liquor becomes desirable, as a means of exciting sensations, and of obviating the irksomeness of having nothing to do.

Inactivity is thus doubly destructive to health. First, by its own primary effects; and, secondly, by leading to intemperance.

Long sittings at meals should be avoided in this climate. All the evils resulting from the sources which have been already mentioned, are increased by the fashionable custom of spending three or four hours at the dinner table, for it leads to them all. The use of segars has the same tendency. They occasion a waste of the saliva, and of course injure the digestion of our food. They produce artificial thirst, and consequently lead to tipling. By taking off that sense of uneasiness which results from having nothing to do, they destroy one of the most powerful incentives to action, and lead to habits of indolence. The smoke of the segars tends to correct the moisture of the atmosphere, and the use of them in some constitutions may advantageously evacuate redundant phlegm; but the small advantages procured in this way are outweighed by many greater evils which flow from their daily use.

Sudden changes from hot to cold air, violent exertions, depressing passions, hard rides, long walks, great fatigue, and excesses of all kinds, should be guarded against by those who are

anxious

anxious for the preservation of health. These cautions are particularly necessary in the interval between June and October; for, during that time, there is such a morbid irritability of the whole system, that irregularities, which in other months of the year might be harmless, seldom fail of immediately drawing after them serious consequences.

Hunting clubs should be wholly discontinued through the summer. They begin with violent exercise, and this is followed by plentiful eating and drinking. After excessive perspiration has been excited by these means, a ride late in the evening closes the scene. Few situations occur in which there is so dangerous a combination of the causes of our fevers as takes place on these occasions. For similar reasons the game of fives, cricket, and in short every species of diversion or exercise that requires violent exertions should be abandoned in warm weather.

The time of exposure to the sun should be shortened as much as possible. While we are necessarily exposed to it, we should abstain from ardent spirits, and should avoid standing still. It would also be proper to protect our heads from the effects of heat, by wearing white hats. These will be much the better for deep crowns on such a construction as leaves a vacancy between the head and the hat. Fashion, which seldoms consults either health or convenience, has lately deviated into what is salutary by introducing the use of flapped hats on the above construction. Long may this fashion

fashion continue, or rather may it never cease to be the fashion in Carolina.

We should be careful of lying in damp rooms, or in linen not sufficiently dry; and we should always put on dry cloaths, as soon as possible, after being wet. Chilling easterly winds, night air, and the evening dews should be avoided. The latter are more pernicious than a thorough wetting from rain. Dew in this climate is of such a penetrating nature, that no ordinary covering can be depended on for excluding it. It insinuates itself through our cloaths, and coming in contact with the skin, checks those discharges which health requires. They who indulge themselves in spending their evenings in open balconies, often pay dear for the hazardous gratification. The ground on which Charleston stands was probably gained from the ocean, and is but a little higher than the ordinary level of the sea. By digging eight or ten feet, we every where find water. From this circumstance, together with the lowness of the ground, and the abundance of swamps and marshes, we breathe an air abounding with moisture. The heat of the sun so commonly but unjustly complained of, is beneficial by correcting this moisture; but when his chearful influence is withdrawn, the natural dampness of the air becomes eminently pernicious. Sleeping with open windows is, for these reasons, very injurious, especially if great changes of the atmosphere take place in the time of sleep. Habit has so far inured several persons to this practice, that they suffer nothing from it.

It

It must also be acknowledged, that the confined air of a small close room soon becomes unfit for respiration. In estimating matters of this kind, the advantages and disadvantages should be weighed against each other. An opinion formed in this way would, as a general rule, be in favor of sleeping with shut windows, especially such as are near our beds. Perhaps the plan most consistent with health and comfort would be, to sleep in a room altogether close, except a door which opened into an adjoining one, into which there was a free admission of the external air. In every case we should so arrange ourselves as to be secure, that wind may not blow directly on us when we are at rest, and especially when we are composed for sleep. The body of a man asleep is in itself considerably cooler than when he is awake. There is, therefore, great danger from that undesigned sleep which often steals upon us in consequence of those lollings in which, when the weather is hot, we are prone to indulge ourselves. They who wish to preserve health should resist all temptations to sleep, except in circumstances where proper precautions are taken for defending the body from that abatement of animal heat which results from sleep itself, and still more from changes of the atmosphere.

The greatest care should be taken for the preservation of cleanliness in our persons, houses, kitchens, yards, stables, pumps and streets. The drains should be kept constantly free from obstructions; but if this cannot be done, the grates over them

them should be covered to keep down the effluvia that would otherwise issue from them to the great danger of the inhabitants. The low grounds of this city, in which water usually stagnates, should be filled up*.

All offensive and putrifying substances should be burnt up, or at least removed, so as to prevent their poisoning the air we breathe. The number of dead animals, and the quantity of putrid vegetables in our streets, is a nuisance of the most dangerous kind. The expence of keeping the city clean would be much less than what is expended in curing the diseases that are fostered by the filth of our streets. The weeds which surround the planters houses in the country should, for the same reason, be burned in that season of the year when they begin to rot.

Costiveness ought to be particularly avoided in this climate. Regularity in the alvine discharges is of the last consequence. Their retention, by disturbing the whole animal œconomy, proves a source of many evils. Whenever these discharges do not return at their proper period, efficacious methods should be immediately adopted to aid the languid bowels in the discharge of their necessary functions. Rising early is one of the best means of obviating costiveness. The cool morning air

tends

---

* This might be done to a considerable extent, with little trouble or expence. If housekeepers would charge themselves with filling up the ponds before their own doors and in their own yards, a saving would soon be made in their Doctors bills which would amply reimburse them.

tends to throw the excrementitious humors on the bowels, and to haſten their diſcharge. The reverſe is the caſe with ſuch perſons as ſpend an undue proportion of their time in a recumbent poſture, and particularly thoſe who lie in bed after ſunriſe. Attention to the ſtate of the bowels is particularly indiſpenſible in the ſummer and firſt months of the autumn. In moſt of the diſeaſes between June and November, the bile is more or leſs injuriouſly predominant, and ſhould be daily diſcharged. In the beforementioned period every article of meat or drink, known by experience to generate a ſurpluſage of bile, ſhould be either wholly laid aſide, or ſparingly uſed; and coſtiveneſs ſhould be obviated by the uſe of laxative food. Perhaps no ſimple in the power of every perſon is more efficacious, in preventing bilious complaints, than raw eggs beat up into an agreeable mixture and taken every morning.

If notwithſtanding all our precautions to the contrary, a fever is beginning to form, inſtead of indulging the vain hope, that it will go off itſelf, we ſhould inſtantly retreat to our chambers, and take ſomething, that by reſtoring an equable perſpiration will turn the current of humors from within outwardly. Nothing does this ſo effectually as a vomit. A proper medicine of that kind taken in time, when the introductory ſymptoms forebode a fever, will often deſtroy it in embryo, prevent a fit of ſickneſs, and the neceſſity of taking a variety of other medicines.

In enumerating what ought to be done to preserve health, the advantages of temperance and exercise are obvious; but instead of dilating on principles suited to every situation, it will be more proper to dwell on such as especially apply to our own. For eight months of the year, South-Carolina is as healthy as any part of the globe. Our winters are delightful, and our greatest summer heats are far from being intolerably distressing. The mercury in the thermometer rises every year as high in Boston, New-York and Philadelphia, as in Charleston. I have lived in both of the latter cities, and can with truth declare, that I have suffered more from heat, in each of them, than I ever did in Charleston. If our summers are longer, and render us less able to bear continued fatigue, this is amply compensated by the superior mildness of our winters and the superior fertility of our soil, which requires less labor for procuring subsistence. The inhabitants of this state are in general, at all times, less liable to rheumatisms, coughs, colds, and inflammatory disorders, than those who live in colder climates. Consumptions, except a few from catarrh, are seldom seen amongst our own citizens. Gravel and stone are comparatively rare in this country. But to fevers of the low kind, we are particularly exposed, especially in the interval between June and November As these may be considered to be the endemic of the country, I beg leave to offer some practical observations on the means of preventing them. Our summer and autumnal fevers, as far as they depend on local situation,

situation, chiefly arife from the feparate or combined influence of heat, moifture, and marfh miafmata. To fecure the body againft the effects of thefe enemies to health, is, or ought to be, an object of general attention. With this view, I would recommend the wearing of flannel next the fkin. It has already been obferved, that in fummer perfpiration is great. Perhaps it is fortunate for us that it is fo, for as many of our humors are by heat rendered morbid, the feafonable difcharge of them is highly beneficial. Where a perfon is immediately covered with linen, the perfpirable matte, as faft as thrown off, is collected and kept in contact with the ducts from which it exuded. On the other hand, flannel, by abforbing the fame, removes much of it from the fkin. As the difcharge of this excrementitious matter is beneficial, the retention of it muft be injurious. The gentle friction of flannel, which foon ceafes to be difagreeable, acts like a flefh brufh, and promotes an agreeable regular perfpiration, than which nothing is more conducive to health. Where the trunk of the body is immediately covered with woollen of any kind, the chance of fuffering from fudden changes of the atmofphere is greatly leffened. Summer colds are infinitely more dangerous than thofe which take place in winter. To thefe we are particularly expofed in the latter end of the warm weather, when the nights begin to grow cool. They who confult only prefent gratification, are apt to difencumber themfelves from the bed cloaths, and in that fituation they go to fleep. This, though harmlefs in

the

the first part of the night, often becomes injurious before day, either from sudden changes of the atmosphere, or from that gradual cooling of it which takes place towards autumn. He who sleeps in flannel has a constant defence against those changes, and is thereby fortified against a common exciting cause of the disorders of the season. Such as cannot reconcile themselves to the wearing of flannel constantly, should at least put it on when they are particularly exposed. The inhabitants of Charleston going to the country when fevers are rife, would do well to observe this precaution, while they are out of the city, especially if their business leads them to be much in rice fields, or in the vicinity of stagnant waters.

Cold bathing, under proper regulations, is an excellent preventive of the diseases of this country. As heat relaxes, it is obvious that cold must brace. Once in twenty-four hours, to immerse the body in cold water, most powerfully strengthens the whole system. Perspiration, though for a moment checked, increases with the returning glow, which immediately follows when the bathed person is wiped dry and begins to take exercise. If this is done in the evening, it seldom fails of procuring a good night's rest; if in the morning, it fortifies the body for bearing the heat of the following day. By bracing the whole system, it destroys that predisposition to diseases, which is brought on by the relaxing qualities of heat and moisture. It is farther serviceable by keeping the skin constantly clean. Such is the excessive perspiration in this country;

country, in the summer, that frequent washings are indispensably necessary to preserve cleanliness. This precaution is too often neglected where periodical bathings are disused. The advantages from even a partial use of the cold bath are great. Colds in the head are very uncommon when it is daily washed in cold water. The eyes of a person who frequently plunges them, wide open, into cold water, will seldom be either weak or inflamed. Diseases of the throat rarely attack those who daily wash their necks with cold water. Frequent washings of the mouth prevent much of the toothache. It has already been observed, that the person who daily washes his feet in cold water, will hardly ever suffer from exposing himself to the dews of the morning. So many diseases might be prevented, and so much good might be done by a judicious use of bathing, that every gentleman ought to have an apparatus in his house for that purpose. Sometimes cold water, and sometimes tepid, ought to be used. In other cases washing would be preferable to bathing. To adjust these, and several other particulars, and to prevent the mischiefs that might arise from indiscreet bathing, the advice of a physician is often necessary.

The aliment used in summer should be antiseptic and generous. The influence of what we eat and drink is very great. Butter and fat meats tend evidently to clog the stomach and vitiate the bile, and therefore should be laid aside, or sparingly used in hot weather. A due proportion of meat and vegetables is proper. Pepper, and the other warm condiments, which are used in seasoning, though in theory they seem to be improper, in a country where heat abounds, are found by experience to be wholesome. They are for the most part the productions of warm climates, and we find that the productions of all countries suit best with their inhabitants. As no dish is more common among negroes than pepperpot, so none is more wholesome. Dr. Lind observes, that " the negroes in the torrid zone commonly mix the most stimulating, poignant sauces with their ordinary light food, and this is experimentally found suitable to their constitutions." In using fruit the following cautions should be observed. It should be thoroughly ripe, and taken only in moderation, and baked or stewed rather than raw. A total abstinence, for some time after recovering from fevers, would be best for convalescents. Watermelons are not only innocent but useful. They may safely be taken in many fevers, and under qualified circumstances, tend to prevent the diseases usually prevalent when they are in season. Water is Nature's diluent. It is the only drink that can be safely taken at all times and by all persons; but, nevertheless, men in every age and country, and in every state of society, have sought for something that was more stimulant. Of all the additions made to water for that purpose, rum is the most pernicious. It contains no nourishment, but like a slow poison insensibly undermines the springs of life. As mankind will not content themselves with nature's beverage, it is the duty of of phyficians to direct them to such substitutes as bring the greatest benefits with the least injury. Of this clafs are liquors which are prepared by fermentation, and also thofe which are expreff'd from vegetables. Of the drinks ufed among us, none are equal to porter and wine for preventing fevers. The former, by its bitternefs, ftrengthens the ftomach, while it proves highly nutritious, and at the fame time moderately evacuant. Obftinate vomitings are fometimes cured by it, more effectually than by the moft celebrated officinal compofitions. Within ten years paft, in which the inhabitants of this city have generally exchanged punch for porter, they have grown much more healthy. Complaints of the bowels have fenfibly leffened. Phyficians are not now called upon to attend one patient with the dry belly-ache for every ten they formerly vifited. Punch, when weak and taken in moderation, and no oftener than occafionally, is falutary and refrefhing, but by no means fuits for common drink. The fame obfervation holds good with refpect to cyder. Mineral acids, diluted with water, correct bile, and refift our fummer difeafes; but this cannot be affirmed of drinks prepared with limes and fuch like vegetable acids when freely and frequently taken. Thefe remarks, though generally well founded, admit of exceptions.

The temperate ufe of good found wine is one of the moft effectual, as well as one of the pleafanteft, antidotes to fevers. It is highly antifeptic, and both prevents and cures putrid difeafes. It is

much

much more worthy of the appellation of a cordial, than any of the boasted officinal compositions, which are called by that name. Different constitutions require different wines, but in general old Madeira agrees best with the inhabitants of Carolina. All physicians know, that in low fevers a liberal use of wine is an essential part of the cure. In order to get the full benefit of this most desirable preventive of our summer diseases, it should not be drank every day. If it was laid aside in the winter and spring, and resumed on the approach of summer, and continued in daily use, only for three or four months, its efficacy in preventing summer and autumnal diseases would be greatly increased. The person who, with the above limitations, drinks from half a pint to a pint of wine every twenty-four hours cannot, in this climate, be justly deemed intemperate.

The daily use of strong warm teas is pernicious. Many respectable medical authorities might be produced, which concur in representing East-India tea as unfriendly to the nerves. Be this as it may, all must acknowledge, that the warm water, which is used as its vehicle, must be unsuitable to this climate.

Cheerfulness is of particular service in preserving health. Many of our diseases flow from bile, and fretfulness never fails to cause an increased flux of that acrid humor into the stomach. Those who watch their own feelings may observe, that when any wayward event breaks in on the peace of their minds, a bitter taste is immediately felt. This
proceeds

proceeds from an overflowing of bile. Bilious persons are for the most part peevish, and peevish persons are for the most part bilious. Bile and fretfulness seem to be reciprocally cause and effect, and both predispose to dangerous disorders. The eyes are sometimes observed to turn suddenly yellow, in a gust of passion. They who are blessed with a constant, equable flow of cheerful spirits, are exempted from one of the occasional causes of fevers: On the other hand, such as give way to peevishness, or to the depressing passions, are particularly exposed to the diseases, which a low, moist country is apt to produce.

In particular habits, the daily use of jesuit's bark, from July till October, is adviseable. Three doses of it, combined with a little rhubarb if necessary, taken in substance, every day or every other day, where ordinary precautions are taken, may in general be relied upon as an effectual antidote to the summer and autumnal fevers of this country.

Throughout the summer and the first month of the autumn, fires are more useful in damp days, than in the dry cold weather of winter. They correct the excessive moisture of the atmosphere, and counteract the exciting causes of the complaints most usual in the before mentioned seasons.

In the construction of our houses, we sacrifice health to profit and convenience, by digging cellars underneath them. The walls at their sides, and covers to their bottoms, lessen the evils that might otherwise result from them, but it would be better if there was not a cellar in the city. The evils

evils arising from this source are of such a magnitude, as to need the interposition of the city council. A law to compel all the inhabitants to pump the water out of their cellars, as soon as it begins to stagnate, would be salutary. It must have frequently occurred to every attentive observer, that, in wet seasons, the cellars in the low part of this city emit such putrid exhalations, as are sensibly offensive even to passengers. They who live over such cellars, or in the vicinity of them, must, therefore, be particularly exposed to diseases, and when sick, are with difficulty cured, unless they remove to a purer atmosphere.

The practice of planting trees before the doors of dwelling houses, is recommended by sound medical reasoning. It has been demonstrated, that trees absorb unhealthy air, and discharge it in a highly purified state, in the form of what modern chymists call dephlogisticated air. It is only to be lamented, that the custom is not universal, and that some uniformity is not observed in the disposition of these beneficial ornaments. Should the present city council make effectual arrangements for planting magnolias, or such like trees, every twelve or fifteen feet, on each side of our streets, through their whole length, they would merit the thanks of the rising generation.

Whether paving the streets of Charleston would conduce to the health of the inhabitants, has been doubted by many. It might add to the heat of the air, but would lessen its morbid qualities, by repressing exhalations. As dry heat alone is a
much

much less evil than heat, moisture and miasmata combined, it is probable, that the inhabitants would be gainers, on balancing the advantages against the disadvantages that would result from paving the streets of this city.

In constructing our city houses, we should endeavor to make them, especially on their north, south and west sides, as open as possible to favor the circulation of fresh air. A man in health pollutes a gallon of air in a minute, to such a degree, as to render it unfit for the purposes of life. The danger of breathing confined, unventilated air, must be therefore self-evident. On these principles, the use of curtains, other than those for excluding musquitoes, may be advantageously dispensed with. They seldom or never do any good, and by confining and heating the air often do harm.

The late practice of adding an attic story to low houses, is not only ornamental but beneficial. It increases the chances for health. The higher we ascend into the atmosphere, the cooler it is, and the farther are we removed from those poisonous exhalations which, though they rise from the earth and stagnant waters, seldom or never ascend to any considerable height. It is on these accounts prudent to sleep in the highest apartments of our houses, unless where their low pitch and converging sides make them warmer than those which are on the lower floors.

Wooden houses are most suitable to this climate. They are much drier, and consequently healthier, than those which are built with brick.

The

The latter abforb and retain, for a long time, much of that moisture with which our atmosphere abounds. The speedy rotting of paper on brick walls proves their dampness. This is particularly the case, when some of their sides are inaccessible to the sun. In such situations they are seldom, for any considerable length of time, thoroughly dry. On this account, such of the inhabitants of this city as are troubled with rheumatic pains, coughs and complaints of the breast, should not live on that part of the Bay which is between its southern extremity and Broad-street. The houses there are mostly built with brick, and are so closely connected together, that two, and often three, of their sides are, for the greatest part of the day, sheltered from the direct rays of the sun. Moisture there predominates, and, in conjunction with easterly winds, is very unfavorable to children and such as have weak lungs. Brick houses would be much drier than they usually are, if a vacancy was left between the walls and the plastering on their insides. This might easily be done by means of studs projecting but a few inches from the walls.

The position of our country houses, with respect to swamps, ought to be attended to; for the summer winds, sweeping along their surface, waft destruction to the inhabitants. In general, the planters would do well to encourage the growing of trees, between their houses and the neighboring swamps; and to construct their houses so as to have neither doors nor windows fronting on marshy ground; but as this cannot always be done, they
should

should build on the south sides of their rice fields and other waters. The winds in the summer months are for the most part southerly. To be under a necessity of breathing air, saturated with the noxious effluvia acquired in passing over stagnant waters, must be highly injurious. Indeed if health was, as it ought to be, preferred to riches, the planters would build their dwelling houses at a distance from the rivers. The inhabitants of a house in the pine barren has a much better chance for health, than he whose mansion is erected in the neighbourhood of any body of water, either stagnant or running. Health and wealth seem to be at variance. The same qualities of the soil which make it fruitful, make it also unwholsome, while the dry surface of pine barren presents comparatively a pure and wholsome air. Besides, the resin of the pine trees in itself contributes to the salubrity of the atmosphere. It is an old and well authenticated observation, that persons, whether white or black, employed in burning tar-kilns, are always healthy. The method practised by Indians and negroes of living in smoke, is conducive to health; but the inconvenience of such a situation will forever operate against its being introduced into common use among our citizens; but, nevertheless, some considerable analogous benefit, with little expence or inconvenience, might be procured to those who reside in the country, from fires kindled round or near their houses. These will be more necessary when the wind is easterly, and more beneficial if made with resinous pine-wood.

On

On these principles, there is no difficulty in accounting why Charleston is more healthy than the neighboring parishes. It has long been observed in low countries, that they who reside in towns, are more healthy than those who live dispersed in the country, and that the inhabitants of the central parts of towns are healthier than those who live in their extremities. The fire and smoke from several hundred contiguous kitchens cannot fail of diminishing the moistness of the atmosphere. The frequent ringing of bells, the flowing of the tides, the motion of carriages and of persons, occasions a brisker circulation of air in this city, than in the adjacent country. The policy of removing, on the approach of summer, from the country to Charleston, is therefore wise. The proper time for making this change varies in different years. In general it may be observed, that it should be early, if a wet spring is followed by a dry summer. While successive rains keep the waters in motion, the danger is little; but when warm and dry weather continues for some time after heavy rains have fallen, fevers will probably soon begin to rage.

Strangers who propose to reside in this country, and our own citizens who have been long absent, when intending to return, should make a point of arriving here about the month of November. They would then have at least half a year to be assimilated to the climate, before their health would be endangered by any thing peculiar to it. The sudden deaths among us of persons disused to our country, are to be referred to an injudicious choice

of

of time for coming to it, and still more to their own imprudence, combined with the hospitality of the inhabitants. To be invited almost daily to the plentiful tables of their friends and acquaintances, is the misfortune of such persons. A fever, rapid in its progress, and fatal in its issue, is frequently the consequence. Strangers coming into this country should be doubly on their guard, but instead thereof they too often suffer themselves to be feasted into fevers, and not unfrequently out of their lives.

On a review of the whole subject, it may be observed, that instead of saying, " this capital is more sickly than the other maritime towns of the United States," it ought only to be said, " that more care is necessary on the part of its inhabitants for the preservation of their health." By proper attention to our children, and especially by steady, discreet management of mothers, much of the mortality of infants might be prevented, and a new generation be reared, which would be much hardier and better adapted to the climate than many of the present. In families where children have been properly brought up, many of both sexes have as good constitutions as are enjoyed by those who live in more northern latitudes. The honors of old age are often attained by our citizens. Indeed the chance of life to a person who is above sixty years old, is considerably in favor of the inhabitants of warm countries. It must be acknowledged, that the variableness and sudden changes of our atmosphere make caution
indispensable;

indispensable; but this as enforcing the necessity of a sober, orderly life, ought to be esteemed an advantage. None of the blessings of this world can be attained without care. It is, therefore, unreasonable to look for health on easier terms. Much attention is necessary to preserve, even a good estate, from running to waste. The same is requisite for guarding a sound constitution against diseases. As well may the planter, who rarely visits his plantation, expect a good crop, as the man who lives at random, look for the continued enjoyment of health. Such as are for a short life and a merry one, must abide by the consequences of their choice. But they who conduct with prudence, and have self-denial to abstain from such practices as experience may have proved to be hurtful, and steadiness to follow what by the same unerring rule they have found to be salutary, may live as healthily, and as long in this city, as in any part of the world.

THE END.

A SKETCH

OF THE

SOIL, CLIMATE, WEATHER,

AND

DISEASES

OF

SOUTH-CAROLINA,

READ BEFORE THE MEDICAL SOCIETY OF THAT STATE,

BY

DAVID RAMSAY, M. D.

VICE-PRESIDENT OF THE SOCIETY.

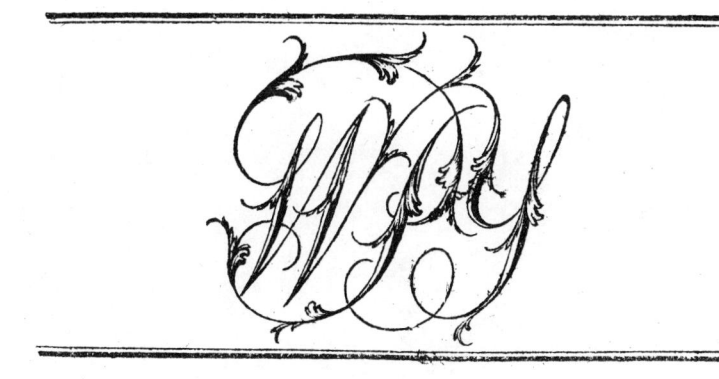

CHARLESTON
PRINTED BY W. P. YOUNG,
FRANKLIN'S HEAD, NO. 43, BROAD-STREET.

MDCCXCVI.

SKETCH

OF THE

SOIL, CLIMATE, WEATHER, AND DISEASES

OF

SOUTH-CAROLINA.

South-Carolina nearly resembles a triangle—It is bounded on the east by the Atlantic ocean, and extends thereon about two hundred miles; on the south, and partly on the west by the river Savannah; and on the north, and partly on the west by North-Carolina. These two last mentioned boundary lines approximate to each other, about three hundred miles from the sea-coast, and in the vicinity of the Alleghany mountains.

The state of South-Carolina lies between the 32d and 35th degrees of north latitude. Its chief city, Charleston, is in north latitude 32° 45, and in west longitude from London, 79°, and from Philadelphia, 5°, and stands on a point of land between the junction of Ashley and Cooper rivers, and about ten miles from the ocean.

In treating of South-Carolina, the philoſopher, as well as the politician, muſt conſider it as divided into upper and lower country. Nature has marked this diſtinction in many particulars. Along the ſea-coaſt, and for one hundred miles weſtward, the country is generally low and flat; from thence, to its weſtern extremity, it is diverſified with hills, riſing higher and higher, till they terminate in the Alleghany mountains, which are the partage ground of the eaſtern and weſtern waters. In the vallies, between theſe hills, a black and deep loam is found. This has been formed by abraſion from the hills, and from rotten trees and other vegetables, which have been collecting for centuries.

The rivers of the upper country originate in the mountains, and are an aſſemblage of ſtreams. After theſe have paſſed into the low country, they move ſlowly, and in a ſerpentine courſe, till they empty into the ocean. The rivers of the low country are, properly, arms of the ſea, extending but a few miles till they head in ſwamps and marſhes.

Carolina, lying on the eaſt ſide of the partage ground, between the eaſtern and weſtern waters, is conſiderably lower than the correſponding parts of the United States, which are on its weſt ſide. Hence it follows, that when the ſnows melt, or heavy rains fall on the mountains, much more of the water,
proceeding

proceeding from thefe fources, is determined to the Atlantic ocean than to the river Miffifipi. In confequence of which, we are often too wet, while our weftern neighbours are too dry.

The fide of South-Carolina, which borders on the fea, is interfected by thirteen rivers, viz. The Waccamaw, Black-river, Santee, Wandow, Cooper, Afhley, Stono, Edifto, Afheppoo, Combahee, Coofaw, Broad, and May rivers. Some of thefe have two mouths, others have feveral heads, or branches. The river Santee, in particular, is formed by a junction of the waters of the Enoree, Tyger, Pacolet, and Catawba rivers, which originate in the mountains. All of the firft mentioned thirteen rivers have a margin of fwamp always on one fide, but often on both, extending from half a mile to three miles.

Thefe fwamps, in their natural ftate, abound with ufeful timber of various kinds, and, when cleared, they reward their cultivators with plentiful crops, efpecially in feafons that are exempt from frefhes. In the intervals between thefe rivers, there are often inland fwamps, frefh-water lakes, and great quantities of low level land, which, after heavy rains, continue for a long time overflowed. The remainder is a dry, and, for the moft part, a fandy foil.

The soil of South-Carolina is naturally, and, for the purposes of taxation, politically divided into the following classes. 1, Tide-swamp. 2, Inland swamp. 3, High river swamp, or low grounds, commonly called second low grounds. 4, Salt marsh. 5, Oak and hickory high land. 6, Pine barren. The tide and inland swamps are peculiarly adapted to the culture of rice and hemp. The high river swamps to hemp, corn, and indigo. The salt marsh has hitherto been, for the most part, neglected; but there is reason to believe, that it would amply repay the expence and labour of preparing it for cultivation. The oak and hickory high land is well calculated for corn and provisions, and also for indigo and cotton. The pine barren is the least productive species of our soil, but it is the most healthy. Daily experience proves that, under certain circumstances, it may be cultivated to advantage for provisions, indigo, and cotton. A proportion of it is an indispensably necessary appendage to a swamp plantation. It is remarkable that ground of this last description, though comparatively barren, affords nourishment to pine trees, which maintain their verdure through winter, and administer more to the necessities and comforts of mankind than any other trees whatsoever. This may perhaps, in part, be accounted for by the well-known observation, that much of the pine land of this state is only superficially sandy, for by digging into it a few inches or feet, the

soil,

soil, in many places, changes from sand to clay.

In digging into the swamps, on the margin of the rivers, the operator frequently meets with the trunks of large trees, which appear to have been buried for ages, and is always arrested in his progress by the springing of water. As deep as these swamps have been penetrated, they consist of a rich blue clay, or a black soft mould, of inexhaustable fertility.

From this description of the low country, it is apparent, that there must be a predominance of moisture; and from the co-operation of heat, there is a strong tendency to putrefaction. From the same causes, and the presence of acid gases, floating in the common atmosphere, metals are very subject to rust. This is particularly the case with iron, which, when exposed to the air, loses, in a short time, all its brightness, and much of its solidity.

The climate of South-Carolina is in a medium between that of tropical countries, and of cold temperate latitudes. It resembles the former in the degree and duration of its summer heat, and the latter in its variableness. In tropical countries, the warmest and coolest days, do not, in the course of a twelve month, vary more from each other than sixteen degrees of Fahrenheit's thermometer: there is,
consequently,

consequently, but little distinction between their summer and winter: but a variation of 83 degrees between the heat and cold of different days in the same year, and of 46 degrees in the different hours of the same day in South-Carolina, is to be found in its historical records.

In our coolest summers, the mercury in the thermometer* has reached 89, and in the five last years in which observations have been made by this society, it has never risen above 93, nor fell below 28. In the year 1785 it stood for a few hours at 96, which was its greatest height since the year 1752, when it rose to 101. In the year 1794 it was never lower than 34, during the time of observation, which began at eight in the forenoon, and ended at ten in the evening. The difference between our coolest and warmest summers, therefore, ranges between 89 and 96; and the difference between our mildest and severest winters, ranges between 34 and 28. Our greatest heat is sometimes less, and never much more, than what takes place in the same season in Baltimore, Philadelphia, and New-York;

* Fahrenheit's thermometer is what is every where meant in this publication, and the observations on it, therein referred to, were reported to the medical society, as taken by Dr. Robert Wilson, at his house, the west end of Broad-street, at the hours of eight in the morning, between two and three in the afternoon, and at ten in the evening. The instrument was suspended in an open passage, about ten feet from the earth.

York; but their warm weather does not, on an average, continue above six weeks, while ours lasts from three to four months. Our nights are also warmer than theirs. The days in Charleston are moderated by two causes, which do not exist, in an equal degree, to the northward of it. Our situation open and near the sea, almost surrounded by water, and not far distant from the torrid zone, gives us a small proportion of the trade winds, which blowing from the south-east are pleasantly cool. These generally set in about 10 A. M. and continue for the remainder of the day. A second reason may be assigned from the almost daily showers of rain that fall in the hottest of our summer months.

Since we began our meteorological journal (January, 1791) the mercury in the thermometer has never been under 28, though in the year 1752 it was down to 18. Mr. Hemitt, in his historical account of South-Carolina, asserts, that he had seen the mercury in Fahrenheit's thermometer, down to 16, and that others had observed it as low as 10. On the whole, for five years past, our greatest heat has been eight degrees, and our greatest cold ten degrees less than they were about the middle of this century, as observed by Dr. Chalmers. A similar observation, though not to the same extent, will result from comparing the greatest heat and cold of the five last years, 1791, 1792, 1793, 1794, and 1795,

1795, as recorded by the medical fociety, with the years 1750, 1751, and 1752, the three firft years recorded by Dr. Chalmers. The greateft heat in 1791, was 90, in 1792, 93, in 1793, 89, in 1794, 91, in 1795, 92; but the greateft heat in 1750, was 96, in 1751, 94, in 1752, 101. The greateft cold in 1791, was 28, in 1792, 30, in 1793, 30, in 1794, 34, in 1795, 29; but in the year 1750, it was 25, in 1751, it was 23, and in 1753, it was 18. Whether this change is accidental, or the confequence of an improvement in our climate, time and future obfervations muft determine. The advantages refulting to the temperature of the air, and to the healthinefs, as well as to the appearance of any country, from the art of man, inhabiting and cultivating it, are inconceivably great. We may, therefore, indulge the hope, that ours is progreffively meliorating from permanent and encreafing caufes.

The quantity of low and moift ground in Carolina, is daily diminifhing. Cultivation naturally tends to exficcation. Wherever the tide flows it brings fomething with it, which being left, helps to fill up cavities. Indeed the furface of the earth naturally, and univerfally, approximates to a level. The rains wafh from the high grounds, and add what is carried away to the low. The bones of an enormoufly large animal have been lately dug up in Biggin-fwamp, by the labourers

bourers at the Santee Canal, eight feet under ground. The trunks of trees have been frequently found at an equal or greater depth. It is possible that these may have been buried below the surface of the ground, as deep as they were lying, but it is much more probable that they originally sunk in the earth, one, two, or three feet, by their own weight, and were afterwards covered by successive alluvions in the lapse of time, to the depth at which they were found.

In proportion as our country has been cleared and cultivated, its rich low grounds, from various causes, have become higher and drier. Much sand and dry clay has been blown on them by high winds. The cutting down of trees has destroyed their perspiration. Many hundred gallons of water are daily issuing from every acre of ground that is fully timbered. The exhalation from the bare surface of the earth exposed to the sun, is much greater than it would be, if the same ground was covered with trees. It is a well known fact, that many old rice fields are now much less productive, than they were thirty years ago. It is probable, that the day is not far distant, when much of the swamp of this state, will be converted into dry arable land, more fit for corn than rice. Though the moisture of the soil has in general decreased, with our increasing cultivation, yet freshes in such of our rivers, as originate in the mountains, have, for some years

years paſt, been higher, and more frequent than uſual.

Theſe are ſerious evils, threatening the deſtruction of ſome of our moſt valuable lands. To inveſtigate the cauſes thereof, is an object well worthy the attention of every friend to Carolina. One reaſon aſſigned for the late increaſe of freſhes is, that the clearing of the upper country opens many ſprings, and gives circulation to much of what would, in a ſtate of nature, be ſtagnant water. By means of drains, made with a view of rendering the ground plantable, the water, which would otherwiſe remain quieſcent, till it was either abſorbed, or evaporated, is conducted to the neareſt ſtream, all of which, ſooner or later, empty into the rivers. It is within the recollection of the old inhabitants of our upper country, that the rivers thereof were, in the days of their youth, much more ſhallow than they are at preſent. If the obſervation already made, " That the tide, wherever it flows, brings ſomething with it, which being left behind, helps to fill up cavities," is well founded, may we not ſuppoſe, that the floods, ruſhing down the rivers from the mountains, meet with obſtructions, yearly increaſing, which retard their courſe to the ocean? If this is one cauſe, among others, of the increaſe of freſhes, the remedy would be to expedite the paſſage of the water from the rivers to the ſea, by multiplying and enlarging their vents,

and

and fhortening their courfe. Whether this is practicable to an extent that would fave all the land adjacent to the rivers, is very doubtful; but it certainly might be effected fo as to fave many plantations, provided the owners would fyftematically co-operate in the execution of a judicious plan, for the more fpeedy difcharge of the fuperfluous water.

The common tides in Afhley and Cooper rivers rife in Charlefton from fix to eight feet; the fpring tides from eight to ten. A common tide, with an eaftwardly wind, is higher than a fpring tide, with a weftwardly wind. The tides in general afcend our rivers about thirty five miles from the ocean, in a direct line. The higheft ground in Charlefton, is between nine and ten feet above the higheft fpring tides. This is to be found in George-ftreet, between Meeting and King ftreets. The next higheft ground is in Harlefton, in Wentworth-ftreet. The next in the weft end of Broad-ftreet, near the theatre. The next in Meeting-ftreet, nearly oppofite the new market.

Earthquakes are fo rare, and fo flight, as not to have been noticed in our hiftorical records. A momentary one, that did no damage, is recollected by fome of our old citizens, as having taken place about the middle of the prefent century. But whirlwinds are more common. Thefe, for the moft part, are confined to narrow limits,

limits, and run in an oblique direction, levelling the loftiest trees that stand in their way.

There are some circumstances which make it probable, that the whole of the low country in Carolina, was once covered by the ocean. In the deepest descent into the ground, neither stones nor rocks obstruct our progress, but every where sand or beds of shells: intermixed with these, at some considerable depth from the surface, petrified fish are sometimes dug up. Oyster shells are found in great quantities, at such a distance from the present limits of the sea-shore, that it is highly improbable they were ever carried there from the places where they are now naturally produced. A remarkable instance of this occurs in a range of oyster-shells extending from Nelson's ferry, on the Santee-river, sixty miles from the ocean, in a south-west direction, passing through the intermediate country, till it crosses the river Savannah, in Burke-county, and continuing on to the Oconee-river, in Georgia. The shells in this range are uncommonly large, and are of a different kind from what are now found near our shores. They are in such abundance, as to afford ample resources for building and agriculture. At the distance of six, eight, or ten feet from the surface, near our sea-coast, water universally springs. A small proportion of sea salt is found in all the well water of this city, and it is probable that the whole of it is obtained by filtration from the ocean, or adjacent rivers. Our

Our country partakes so much of the nature of a West-India climate, as to be liable to hurricanes, but these have been less frequent than formerly. Within the first fifty-two years of the present century, three took place, viz. in 1700, 1728, and 1752, but for the last forty-three years nothing of the kind, worthy of notice, has occurred. Our elder citizens inform us, that thunder storms were, in the days of their youth, much more frequent and more injurious than they have been for the last thirty years. This is remarkably the case in Charleston, and is probably, in part, owing to the multiplication of electrical rods. Mr. Hewitt, who wrote about twenty-five years ago asserts, that he had known in Charleston five houses, two churches, and five ships struck with lightning, during one thunder storm. Nothing comparable to this has occurred for many years past. It is nevertheless true, that during the summer, there are few nights, in which lightning is not visible in some part of the horizon.

The transitions from heat to cold are great, and sometimes very sudden. Dr. Chalmers states, that on the 10th of December, 1751, the mercury in Fahrenheit's thermometer fell forty-six degrees in sixteen hours, that is, from 70 to 24. The greatest variation that has taken place in a day, in the five years that have passed since the institution of this society, was on the 28th of October, 1793, when it fell to

37 from 74, at which it ſtood on the 27th; that is thirty-ſeven degrees in the courſe of twenty-four hours.

The number of extreme warm days in Charleſton is ſeldom above thirty in a year, and it is rare for three of theſe to follow each other. On the other hand, eight months out of twelve are moderate and pleaſant. The number of piercing cold days in winter is more, in proportion to our latitude, than of thoſe which are diſtreſſingly hot in ſummer, but of theſe more than three rarely come together. There are, on an average, in this city, about twenty nights in a twelvemonth, in which the cloſeneſs and ſultrineſs of the air forbid us, in a great meaſure, the refreſhment of ſound ſleep, but this ſevere weather is, for the moſt part, ſoon terminated by refreſhing and cooling ſhowers. April, May, and June are, in common, our healthieſt months; Auguſt and September the moſt ſickly; April and May the drieſt; June, July, and Auguſt the wetteſt; November the pleaſanteſt. In ſome years January, and in others February is the coldeſt month. It is remarkable, that when orange trees have been deſtroyed by froſt, it has always been in the month of February. December is the beſt month in the year for ſtrangers to arrive in this city: ſuch ſhould calculate ſo as not to make their firſt appearance either in ſummer, or the two firſt months of autumn. The hotteſt day of the year is

ſometimes

sometimes as early as June, which was the case in the year 1791; sometimes as late as September as in the year 1793; but oftenest in July or August. The hottest hour of the day in Charleston varies with the weather: it is sometimes as early as ten in the forenoon, but most commonly between two and three in the afternoon.

In the spring when the sun begins to be powerful, a langour and drowsiness is generally felt, respiration is accelerated, and the pulse becomes quicker and softer. Strangers are apt to be alarmed at these feelings, and anticipate an increase of them, with the increasing heat of the season, but they find themselves agreeably disappointed. The human frame so readily accommodates itself to its situation, that the heat of June and July is, to most people, less distressing than the comparatively milder weather of April and May. On the other hand, though September is cooler than the preceeding months, it is more sickly, and the heat of it more oppressive. Perspiration is diminished and frequently interrupted; hence the system, debilitated by the severe weather of July and August, feels more sensibly, and more frequently, a sense of languor and lassitude. Besides the coolness of the evenings in September, and the heavy dews that then fall, multiply the chances of getting cold. It is, on the whole, the most disagreeable month in the year.

Frosts

Frosts seldom extend into the ground more than two inches in the coldest seasons. They generally commence about the middle of October, and terminate in the month of March. On their approach they bring with them a cure for the fevers then usually prevalent. The inhabitants of Charleston keep fires in their houses from four to six months in the year, but there are some warm days in every month, in which fires are disagreeable. On the other hand, there are some moist cool days in every month of the year, with the exception of July and August, in which fires are not only healthy but pleasant. Ice is seldom half an inch thick, and rarely gives an opportunity for the wholesome exercise of skating.

The annual medium temperature of the air in Charleston, was $65\frac{2}{12}$ in 1791, 65 in 1792, $65\frac{2}{12}$ in 1793, 65 in 1794, $64\frac{5}{12}$ in 1795. The average medium for these five years, without fractions, is 65. The average medium of the ten years, viz. from 1750 to 1759, which were observed and recorded by Dr. Chalmers, was 66. From these facts it appears probable, that the aggregate heat of different years, in the same place, is nearly equal. A very warm summer is preceeded or followed by a proportionably cold winter, so as to bring different years nearly to the same temperature of the air, on an average of the whole four seasons.

The greatest, least, and mean heat, for every month of the year, for the five last years, will appear from the annexed table.

TABLE OF THE GREATEST, LEAST, AND MEAN DE-
GREES OF HEAT, IN CHARLESTON, FOR THE YEARS

Month.	1791	1792	1793	1794	1795
January	G. 65 L. 35 M. 50	G. 66 L. 30 M. 48	G. 67 L. 36 M. 51½	G. 65 L. 35 M. 50	G. 60 L. 33 M. 46½
Febru.	G. 69 L. 35 M. 52	G. 68 L. 30 M. 49	G. 74 L. 35 M. 54½	G. 70 L. 34 M. 52	G. 63 L. 29 M. 46
March	G. 78 L. 42 M. 60	G. 74 L. 41 M. 57½	G. 72 L. 34 M. 53	G. 76 L. 43 M. 59½	G. 73 L. 33 M. 53
April	G. 82 L. 52 M. 67	G. 80 L. 52 M. 66	G. 83 L. 56 M. 69½	G. 74 L. 50 M. 62½	G. 78 L. 53 M. 65½
May	G. 87 L. 61 M. 74	G. 84 L. 64 M. 74	G. 83 L. 62 M. 72½	G. 86 L. 63 M. 74½	G. 84 L. 70 M. 77
June	G. 87 M. 69 L. 78	G. 89 L. 63 M. 76½	G. 86 L. 70 M. 78	G. 91 L. 65 M. 78	G. 86 L. 71 M. 78½
July	G. 89 L. 66 M. 77½	G. 93 L. 70 M. 81½	G. 88 L. 76 M. 82	G. 85 L. 72 M. 78½	G. 92 L. 74 M. 83
Auguſt	G. 90 L. 74 M. 82	G. 92 L. 69 M. 80½	G. 87 L. 70 M. 78½	G. 91 L. 75 M. 83	G. 88 L. 72 M. 80
Sept.	G. 87 L. 61 M. 74	G. 85 L. 60 M. 72½	G. 89 L. 69 M. 79	G. 88 L. 66 M. 77	G. 83 L. 59 M. 71
Oct.	G. 83 L. 50 M. 66½	G. 77 L. 46 M. 61½	G. 82 L. 35 M. 58½	G. 75 L. 47 M. 61	G. 79 L. 48 M. 63½
Novem.	G. 72 L. 40 M. 56	G. 74 L. 45 M. 59½	G. 76 L. 39 M. 57½	G. 74 L. 37 M. 55½	G. 75 L. 42 M. 58½
Decem.	G. 63 L. 28 M. 45½	G. 70 L. 34 M. 52	G. 66 L. 30 M. 48	G. 68 L. 37 M. 52½	G. 71 L. 30 M. 50½

The evils that every year take place, more or less, in Philadelphia, from drinking cold water, are unknown in this city. Our water lies so near the surface of the earth, that the difference of its temperature from that of the common air, is not so great as to create danger, unless in very particular circumstances. A solitary case occured in September, 1791, of a negro fellow, who, after taking a draught of cold water, when very warm, suddenly fainted away, and, immediately after, became insane, and continued so for several days, but he afterwards recovered.

Instead of sudden deaths from cold water, we have to lament the same event from the intemperate use of spirituous liquors. The stimulus of ardent spirits, added to the stimulus of excessive heat, drives the blood forcibly on the brain, and produces fatal consequences. These are oftener apoplexies than strokes of the sun. Four sots expired suddenly, in one hot day last summer, in one square of this city.

The east and noth-east winds in winter and spring, are very injurious to invalids, especially to those who have weak lungs, or who are troubled with rheumatic complaints. In these seasons they bring with them that languor, for which they are remarkable in other countries; but in summer, by moderating heat, they are rather wholsome than otherwise.

Weft and north-weft winds, which blow over large tracts of marsh, are, in the summer seafon, unfriendly to health. The north and north-weft winds are remarkable for their invigorating effects on the human frame. South winds are healthy in summer, but much less so in winter.

The general direction of the winds in this city, for four succeffive years, may be learnt from the annexed table.

On December 31, 1790, at four o'clock, A. M. wind N. E. a severe snow ftorm began in Charlefton, which continued for twelve hours, in confequence of which, the ftreets were covered with snow, from two to four inches deep, and the sea iflands, north-eaftward, to the depth of six inches. Another took place on the 28th of February, 1792, wind N. W. which continued for several hours, and till it covered the ground five or six inches. These were rare phænomena. Snow is more common, and continues longer in proportion as we recede from the sea-fhore. The further we proceed weftward, till we reach the mountains, which divide the weftern from the eaftern waters, the weather is colder, and vegetation later. While the inhabitants of Charlefton can scarcely bear to be covered, in the hours of fleep, with a fheet, they who live in the town of Columbia, one hundred and twenty miles to the north-weft of

TABLE of the COURSE of the WINDS.

Month.	1791 Wind.	Days	1792 Wind.	Days	1793 Wind.	Days	1794 Wind.	Days
January	N. E. & E. S. W. & W. N. W.	7 3 1	W. & N. W. S. W. N. E.	13 2 15	N. W. & W. S. E. & E. S. W. & S. N. E. & E.	18 4 8 6	N. W. N. E. W. & S. W.	9 10 19
February	S. E. S. W. & W. N. E. & E. N. W.	3 9 12 4	W. & N. W. S. W. N. E. & E.	15 4 11	N. E. & N. N. W. & W. S. E. & E. S. W. & S.	7 12 8 7	N. E. N. W. S. W. & W.	6 11 10
March	N. E. & E. S. W. S. & W. N. W.	12 14 2	W. & S. W. N. W. N. E. & E. S. E.	12 6 5 3	N. E. & E. S. W. & W. N. W. & N. S. E.	9 17 6 7	S. W. & W. S. E. & S. N. W. & N. N. E. & N.	13 11 4 11
April	S. E. & S. S. W. & W. N. E. & E.	5 14 14	S. E. & E. S. W. & W. N. W.	4 21 2	N. E. & E. S. E. & S. S. W. & W. N. W. & N.	14 5 13 4	N. E. & E. S. W. & W. N. W. S. E. & S.	14 3 5 10
May	N. W. & W. S. W. & W. S. E. & E. S. W.	4 12 15 1	W. & S. W. N. N. E. & E. S. E. & E.	13 12 3	S. E. & E. S. W. & W. N. E. N. W.	14 9 10 2	N. E. & N. S. E. & S. S. W. & W. N. W.	10 15 12 7
June	S. E. & E. S. W. & W. N. E.	10 14 2	S. W. & W. S. E. & E. N. E. N. W.	13 10 9 2	S. W. & W. N. S. E. & S.	17 1 4	N. W. & W. S. E. & E. S. W. & S. N. E.	14 7 18 3
July	S. W. & W. N. W. & N. N. E. & E. S. E.	12 3 14 3	S. W. & W. N. E. & E. S. E. N. W.	13 16 7 1	S. W. & W. S. E & S. N. W. N. E. & E.	21 13 2 5	N. E. & E. S. E. & S. S. W. & W. N. W. & N.	7 5 20 2
August	W. S. W. & S. S. E. & E. N. E. N. W.	19 6 2 3	W. & S. W. N. E. & E. S. E. N. W.	12 15 5 4	S. W. N. E. & E. N. W. S. E. & S.	14 11 2 11	N. E. & E. S. W. & W. N. W. & W. S. E. & S.	16 11 3 10
September	S. W. & W. N. W. S. E. & S. N. E.	12 6 6 8	N. E. & E. S. E. & S. S. W. & W. N. W.	23 1 6 3	S. W. & S. S. E. & E. N. E. N. W.	9 10 19 5	N. E. & E. S. E. & S. S. W. & W. N. W.	14 8 15 2
October	N. N. E. & E. N. W. & W. S. E.	16 14 3	N. W. & N. S. W. & W. N. E. & E.	7 4 18	N. E. & E. N. W. & W. S. E. & S. S. W.	20 7 10 4	N. E. & N. N. W. & W. S. E. & E. S. W.	19 5 10 4
November	N. W. N. N. E. S. & S. E.	12 3 7 2	N. W. & W. S. W. & S. N. E. & E. S. E.	18 7 10 8	S. W. & W. N. E. & E. S. E. & S. N. W. & N.	10 10 6 3	S. W. & W. N. E. & E. S. E. N. W.	9 13 2 8
December	W. N. W. & N. N. E. S. W. S. E.	22 3 3 3	N. E. & E. N. W. & N. S. W. & W. S. E.	10 15 11 1	N. W. N. E. & E. S. W. & W. N.	13 5 9 4	N. W. & N. S. W. & W. N. E. & E. S. E. & S.	10 10 10 3

To face p. 18.

SOUTH-CAROLINA.

of it, are not incommoded with a blanket. The difference is greater as we advance to Ninety-fix, Pinckney, and Washington diftricts.

The sum total of rain, on an average of ten years, viz. from 1750 to 1759, as observed by Dr. Chalmers, was 41.75 inches in the year. The quantity of rain that fell in each month of the year 1795, was as follows:

	INCHES.	10ths.
January,	8	5
February,	1	8
March,	4	6
April,	2	4
May,	8	1
June,	8	1
July,	5	2
Auguft,	9	4
Sept. and October,	8	9
November,	0	9
December,	5	0
	71	8 in the year.

In the four years preceeding 1795, before we began to meafure the quantity of rain, the number of days on which it fell in confiderable quantities, without noticing flight tranfient fhowers, was as follows:

DAYS OF RAIN.

	1791	1792	1793	1794
January,	2	12	12	9
February,	8	7	9	5
March,	9	8	11	12
April,	6	2	9	7
May,	3	6	14	8
June,	15	9	8	13
July,	10	9	10	23
Auguft,	10	10	15	13
September,	10	6	8	9
October,	8	4	3	8
November,	9	5	9	10
December,	6	10	6	11
	96	88	114	118

When the waters are kept in motion by a fucceffion of fhowers, it is generally healthy; but fevers are ufually rife, when a feries of warm dry days follows great falls of rain. The ciftern water of this city, collected from rain, is a degree and a half warmer than the well water; and the temperature of the well water is $64\frac{1}{2}$, which is twelve degrees warmer than that of Philadelphia.

Our

Our old people are ofteneft carried off in cold weather; the young, the intemperate, and the labouring part of the community, when it is hot.

It is to be regretted, that bilious remitting and intermitting fevers have increafed in the country, with the clearing thereof. The felling of trees, and opening of avenues to the rivers, have given more extenfive circulation to marfh miafmata. The increafe of mill-dams in the upper country has been injurious to the health of its inhabitants. In Charlefton a change has taken place much for the better. Bilious remitting autumnal fevers have, for fome years paft, evidently decreafed. The fmall-pox is now a trifling diforder, compared with what it was in 1760 and 1763. Pleurifies, which were formerly common and dangerous, are now comparatively rare, and fo eafily cured, as often to require no medical aid. The dry belly-ache has, in a great meafure, difappeared: perhaps this may be in part owing to the increafing difufe of punch. April and May ufed to be the terror of parents; but the difeafes, which thirty years ago occafioned great mortality among children in the fpring, have, for fome years paft, been lefs frequent and lefs mortal. It is now found, by happy experience, that they are often cured, or prevented, by country air. The three laft Aprils have paffed over without any notice being taken on our journals, of

the

the diarrhæa of infants, as having occurred in the practice of the members of this society.

A species of sore throat, accompanied with symptoms of the croup, which formerly swept off numbers of children, has, for the four last years, rarely occurred in practice. More rational methods of treating wives and mothers, have been substituted in lieu of the enervating confinement, imposed in the days of our fathers. The good effects of which are visible in the diminished number of women who die in childbirth, and in the increasing number of children who are now raised to maturity.

Dr. Mosely, in his treatise on tropical diseases, observes as follows, "Hot climates are indeed very favorable to gestation and parturition. Difficult labours are not common, and children are generally born healthy and strong, and thrive more than they do in temperate climates, for a few years, and are not subject to the rickets nor the scrophula." As a proof of this general position, applied to our state, I observe, that, in many instances, from seven to ten, and in a few, from ten to fifteen children have been raised to maturity in South-Carolina, from a single pair. There are now eight families in Broad-street, between the state-house and the western extremity of that street, in which sixty-nine children have been born, and of these fifty-six are alive. In that part

part of Meeting-street, which lies between Tradd-street and Ashley-river, from six marriages, (which, with the exception of one, have taken place since the year 1782) forty-two children have been born, all of which, except three, are now alive, and the eldest of the whole is little more than fourteen. Within the same limits, seven other couple have fifty-two children living, the youngest of whom is twelve years old, and forty-seven are grown to maturity.

Greater instances of fœcundity frequently occur in our middle and upper country, chiefly among those who inhabit poor land, at a distance from the rivers. There is a couple in Orangeburgh district, near the road that leads to Columbia from Orangeburgh, who lately had fifteen children alive out of sixteen, and a fair prospect of more. Another couple live in Darlington-county, fifteen miles from Lynch's-creek, who lately had thirteen children, and fifty-one grand children, all alive; and of their thirteen children, twelve were married at the same time.

The yellow fever raged in this city in the years 1700, 1732, 1739, 1745, 1748; but since the last mentioned year, nothing of the kind, of serious consequence,* has taken place, except

* Some persons die almost every year, with the bilious fever, whose skin is yellow before or after death, and

except the malignant fever of 1792 and 1794; which, though it resembled the yellow-fever in many things, was entirely different in two important particulars. It was not contagious, nor did it affect any person who had, for any considerable time, been used to the air of Charleston.

Sundry persons from the country were infected with it in this city, who died on or immediately after their return; but in no instance was the disease propagated from them, nor among the attendants on those who had the disease in Charleston. It was a fever sui generis, but resembled the typhus icterodes of Sauvage. The whole mortality from it, in 1792 and 1794, did not exceed one hundred and fifty in each year.*

Camp and some of whom discharge black matter by vomiting; but this is very different from what is commonly meant by the West-India yellow-fever.

* It is much to be regretted that regular bills of mortality are not kept in Charleston. To remedy this defect, on a particular occasion, the sextons of the different churches were desired to give information of the number of persons buried in their respective burial grounds, from which it appeared to the medical society, that between the first of August, 1792, and the 26th of October, of the same year, one hundred and sixty-eight white persons were interred in the different burial grounds in Charleston. When it is considered, that the typhus icterodes began about the middle of July, and did not disappear till the middle of October, of this same year, 1792,

February	Catarrhal fevers. Small-pox. Measles. Anginas.	Catarrhal and rheumatic fevers. Scarlatina anginosa.	Catarrhal and rheumatic fevers. Scarlatina anginosa.	Small-pox. Hooping-cough. Catarrhal fevers. Anginas.	Catarrhal and miliary fevers. Measles.
March	Small-pox. Measles.	Catarrhal fevers. Small-pox. Measles. Angina ulcerosa.	Catarrhal fevers. Anginas. Small-pox. Dysentery.	Small-pox. Anginas. Catarrhal fevers. Hooping-cough.	Catarrhal and miliary fevers. Measles.
April	Small-pox. Measles. Diarrhœa of Infants. Scarlatina anginosa.	Small-pox. Measles. Diarrhœa of infants.	Small-pox. Measles. Diarrhœa of infants.	Miliary fevers. Small-pox. Measles. Dysentery.	Measles. Catarrhal fevers. Pleurisies.
May	Small-pox. Measles. Angina ulcerosa. Diarrhœa of Infants.	Small-pox Measles. Hooping cough. Cholera morbus. Dysentery of infants.	Small-pox. Anginas. Hooping-cough. Catarrhal fevers. Dysentery.	Small-pox. Hooping-cough. Bilious remittent and intermittent fevers.	Measles. Catarrhal fevers. Pleurisies. Diarrhœa.
June	Small-pox. Measles. Dysentery. Diarrhœa. Intermittent fevers.	Small-pox. Measles. Dysentery. Intermittent fevers.	Small pox. Diarrhœa. Dysentery. Hooping-cough. Intermittent fevers. Anginas.	Intermittent fevers. Diarrhœa. Dysentery. Small-pox. Hooping cough.	Hooping-cough. Diarrhœa. Dysentery. Intermittent fevers.
July	Small-pox. Measles. Dysentery. Diarrhœa. Intermittent fevers. Scarlatina anginosa.	Small-pox. Dysentery. Measles. Intermittent fevers. Scarlatina.	Small-pox. Hooping-cough. Intermittent fevers. Mumps.	Typhus icterodes. Small-pox. Dysentery and diarrhœa of infants. Hooping-cough.	Small-pox. Hooping-cough. Intermittent fevers. Dysentery. Measles.
August	Bilious intermittent & remittent fevers. Small-pox. Catarrhal fevers. Dysentery and Diarrhœa. Measles.	Typhus icterodes. Catarrhal fevers. Rheumatisms. Small-pox. Measles.	Hooping-cough. Intermittent fevers. Dysentery. Diarrhœa.	Small-pox. Hooping-cough. Diarrhœa and dysentery. Typhus icterodes.	Fevers. Dysentery. Hooping-cough.
September	Intermittent fevers. Catarrhal fevers. Measles. Angina ulcerosa. Croup.	Typhus icterodes. Catarrhal and rheumatic fevers. Dysentery. Hooping cough.	Catarrhal fevers.	Typhus icterodes. Intermittent fevers.	Typhus icterodes. Rheumatic fevers.
October	Catarrhal fevers. Spasmodic colics. Intermittent fevers. Measles.	Intermittent fevers. Croup. Small-pox.	Catarrhal fevers. Scarlatina. Intermittent fevers.	Typhus icterodus. Catarrhal and intermittent fevers. Hooping-cough.	Typhus icterodes. Catarrhal and intermittent fevers.
November	Croup. Scarlatina anginosa.	Small-pox. Hooping-cough. Intermittent fevers.	Hooping-cough. Catarrhal fevers.	Measles. Catarrhal fevers. Anginas. Intermittent fevers. Quinsy.	Typhus icterodes. Intermittent and catarrhal fevers.
December	Measles. Angina ulcerosa. Pleurisies. Catarrhal fevers.	Intermittent fevers. Angina ulcerosa. Catarrhal fevers. Dysentery. Small-pox.	Hooping-cough. Intermittent and Catarrhal fevers.	Measles. Catarrhal fevers.	Catarrhal fevers.

JANUARY.	Catarrhal fevers. Anginas.	Catarrhal fevers. Measles.	Catarrhal and inter-mittent fevers. Angina ulcerosa.	Catarrhal fevers. Hooping-cough.	Measles. Catarrhal fevers.
	1791.	1792.	1793.	1794.	1795.

A TABLE of the Diseases that occurred in Charleston, from 1791, to 1795, in the practice of the Members of the Medical Society, and entered by them on their Journal.

Camp fevers were, as ufual, attendant on the armies in the time of the late war. The fcarlatina anginofa was alfo common in Charlefton, in the year 1783, but attended with little mortality. The typhus icterodes of 1792 and 1794 was confined to ftrangers, and did not extend beyond the limits of this city. Thefe difeafes were, in a limited fenfe, epidemic; but, except the influenza, no ferious extenfive epidemic has taken place among us for the laft twenty years.

The annexed table, extracted from the journals of the medical fociety, will fhew, at one view, the general tenor of the difeafes that have occurred in Charlefton, for the five laft years.

It muft be highly agreeable to every benevolent mind, that Charlefton is now more healthy than formerly, and likely to be more and more fo. With pleafure I anticipate, that in the courfe of the next century, our buildings will be extended into Afhley and Cooper rivers, as far as low water mark; that the adjacent marfhes will be banked in; the ftreets paved, and well provided with fewers; the bogs drained; the low grounds filled up; and the whole area of the city be firm, folid, high, and

1792, and that Auguft and September are the moft fickly months of the whole twelve, the death of one hundred and fixty-eight perfons, in the courfe of eighty-feven days, in a city, whofe white population was about eight thoufand perfons, muft be deemed very moderate.

and dry land. Those who recollect the time when ducks were shot in a pond, which occupied the ground on which the state-house is erected—when a creek ran up to Church-street, and was crossed on a bridge, near where the French church now stands—when they used to swim over that spot of ground which is now Mr. Allston's garden—when Water-street, which, at present, is high and dry, was almost impassable, will acquit me of being too sanguine, when I indulge the hope, that our grand-children will be less exposed to fevers than we are.

It is a glorious exploit in a country, whose maladies chiefly arise from heat and moisture, to redeem its metropolis from moisture, which, of the two, is the most plentiful source of disease. Whoever builds a house, fills a pond, or drains a bog, deserves well of his country.*

It

---

* Our fellow-citizen, Captain Toomer, is entitled to praise on this account; he has converted a very miry spot in Meeting street, into solid ground, and covered it with houses. Much remains to be done in this way, to improve the health of Charleston. The existence of a pond in a city, is a reproach to its police. Efficient measures should be immediately adopted to drain or fill up the low grounds. The streets should be paved, and the sewers constructed on a different plan. They ought to be completely covered over, and extended on each side to the nearest river: while smaller ones, from every house, should enter them near their top, and on a descent. All offensive matter should be transmitted through these lateral sewers to the main one in the middle of the street;
and

It is no small advantage to the inhabitants of Charleston, that they can, in the space of two hours, parry the heat of summer, by going to Sullivan's-island, where many invalids, especially children, have found a speedy restoration to health and strength. Our citizens have gained so much by frequenting this island, we may well wonder that is only three years since it began to be a place of summer resort.

Intermitting fevers are common to those who inhabit on or near to the banks of our rivers. On the other hand, by removing into the high and dry lands, three or four miles from the rivers, ponds, and mill-dams, fevers may, for the most part, be avoided. Of this a remarkable instance has lately occurred in St. Stephens, the inhabitants of which by quitting the swamps in summer, and fixing themselves in a new settlement, called by them Pine-Ville, have, for two years past, in a great measure, escaped the diseases which are common in the most sickly season of the year.

The swamps of South-Carolina terminate about one hundred and ten miles from the sea-coast; from thence westward the country becomes more hilly: the inhabitants are more ruddy, and in general more healthy.

The

and the whole so constructed, that as often as it rained, there would be a general purification of the city.

The tetanus is more common here than in colder countries. Twenty-one cases of it, and most of them fatal ones, have been reported to the medical society, between September, 1791, and August, 1795: seven of these took place in winter. Chronic complaints are comparatively rare in this state. The gravel, the stone, the dropsy, the rheumatism, and the consumption occur much seldomer with us[*] than with our northern brethren. Fevers are our proper endemick: he who escapes them has little else to fear. And much may be successfully done for the avoidance of them by prudent careful active persons, who study their constitutions, and observe a generous medium between living too high and living too low.

Were it possible exactly to contrast the consumptions of New-England with the fevers of South-Carolina, the inhabitants of both would have nearly equal reason to be satisfied with the place of their nativity. As to long life our eastern brethren have the advantage of us. In proportion to numbers, as far as history

---

[*] "In tropical countries, people are seldom affected with dangerous pulmonic diseases; idiotism and mania are very uncommon: lunacy is almost unknown: scurvy and gravel are diseases seldom to be met with, and the stone scarcely ever. I have known many Europeans subject to the gravel at home who had no symptoms of it during their residence in the West Indies."

Mosely on the diseases of tropical climates, p. 112.

tory and obfervation warrant a comparifon, there are as many of their inhabitants reach 85 as of ours who attain to 70.

Extreme old age, though not common, is fometimes attained by our citizens, efpecially by thofe who, in middle or early life, have migrated from the cold northern countries of Europe. A native of this city now refides in it, at Amen corner, who is fuppofed by herfelf and acquaintances, to be an hundred years old. I have been well informed of feven or eight others in different parts of the ftate, who have reached, and in fome cafes exceeded that period. A particular cenfus of the aged inhabitants of this city was taken by Captain Jacob Milligan, in the year 1790, at the requeft of a worthy citizen, fince dead, from which it appeared that there were then, in Charlefton, 198 white perfons who were fixty years of age, and one hundred of thefe were upwards of 70, and one 108. Our white population, at that period, was about 8000.

This imperfect fketch of the foil, climate, weather, and difeafes of South-Carolina, collected from our medical journal, my own obfervations for 22 years, and the information of others, is refpectfully fubmitted to the fociety, with a requeft that each member would freely point out wherein I am deficient, and
where

where I am mistaken. He who, in the spirit of candor and philosophy, corrects me in an old error, or furnishes me with a new truth, deserves, and shall receive my most grateful acknowledgements.

David Ramsay.

CHARLESTON, S. C.
May 1, 1796.

COPY-RIGHT SECURED ACCORDING TO LAW.

AN EXAMINATION INTO THE HEALTH AND LONGEVITY OF THE SOUTHERN SEA PORTS OF THE UNITED STATES WITH REFERENCE TO THE SUBJECT OF LIFE INSURANCE

J[osiah] C. Nott

SOUTHERN JOURNAL

OF

MEDICINE AND PHARMACY.

Vol. II.   CHARLESTON, (S. C.) MARCH, 1847.   No. 2.

ART. I.—*An Examination into the Health and Longevity of the Southern Sea Ports of the United States, with reference to the subject of Life Insurance.* By J. C. NOTT, M. D., of Mobile, Ala.

[CONCLUDED.]

THOUGH the climates and diseases of the Southern Atlantic and Gulf States are not identical, they are made to approximate so nearly *in the cities,* that we may assume identity for our present purposes. Acclimation in one of these climates, gives immunity against the diseases of the others. The inhabitants of Charleston, Savannah, Pensacola, Mobile and New-Orleans, are known to be as safe in one of these towns as another from febrile diseases. I beg therefore it will be remembered, that when I speak generally, or speak of Charleston, my remarks apply to all these places. I have taken the facts which I shall use in illustration of our subject, almost exclusively from the last named city, because it is the only one whose statistics have been kept for any length of time with accuracy, and because the population has been peculiarly stationary, and little disturbed by emigration and immigration, while the others have been greatly acted on by these influences.

I shall now proceed to give with some detail, the statistics of this city and the deductions I have made from them. The statistics, as far as they go, may be as fully relied on, as any records of this kind, and cannot fail to be acceptable to those who take interest in vital statistics.

I have before me a "*Report of the Interments in the City of Charleston, with the name and number of each disease, from* 1828 *to* 1846 (*eighteen years,*) *the prevailing diseases in each month, and thermometrical range, &c., from* 1834 *to* 1846 (*twelve years.*") By John L. Dawson, M.D. City Register.

I have, also, (kindly furnished me by one of the editors of this Journal, from the city records,) the bills of mortality for

122 *Longevity in reference to Life Insurance.*

the last six years, with more full details, which enable me for this period, to give the ages at death, mortality of the different periods of life, &c.

There are very many important details wanting, which I deeply regret, and must console myself by making the best use I can of those we have. As an indispensable preliminary, I will here give the population of Charleston, at several decennial periods, from 1790 to 1840.

POPULATION OF CHARLESTON FROM 1790 TO 1840.

	Whites.	Colored.	Total.
1830—	12,928	17,361	30,289
1840—	13,030	16,231	29,261
	102 increase.	1,130 decrease.	1,028 decrease.

Longevity in reference to Life Insurance.

It will be seen from this table, that the population has been almost stationary for the last eighteen years. The white population between 1830 and 1840, gained but 102, while the colored lost 1130. There could not during this time, have been much immigration, but considerable emigration of both classes, to have kept the population down to these points, otherwise, the natural increase would have added largely to it. I have separated as far as possible, in my calculations, the two castes, but the tables will only permit it in the total mortality of each. The diseases, ages, &c., are all thrown together by the Register. We give below his table of the gross mortality for each year.

	Males.	Females.	Total.	Blk. & Col'd.	Prop'n of Deaths to Population.
1828,	454	339	793	435	one in 37.81
1829,	388	374	762	455	do. 38.14
1830,	408	355	763	434	do. 39.31
1831,	382	351	733	455	do. 41.00
1832,	303	257	560	310	do. 53.57
1833,	281	261	542	306	do. 55.35
1834,	350	342	692	384	do. 43.77
1835,	365	299	664	363	do. 45.55
1836,	639	533	1172	853	do. 25.84
1837,	352	278	630	356	do. 48.00
1838,	828	381	1209	500	do. 25.05
1839,	502	354	856	422	do. 35.38
1840,	261	244	605	348	do. 49.52
1841,	336	258	594	335	do. 50.44
1842,	307	253	560	360	do. 54.47
1843,	368	329	697	483	do. 44.59
1844,	282	271	553	365	do. 54.18
1845	272	298	570	324	do. 52.18

This table is a very important one when taken in connection with other explanatory facts, but by itself is calculated to lead to very erroneous conclusions. It will be made to appear in the sequel, that little fluctuation has occurred in the annual mortality of the *native or acclimated* population, during these eighteen years, and that the great mortality of certain years was from the endemic diseases of the climate which confine their ravages almost exclusively to the *unacclimated*. The year 1836 it appears, was particularly fatal to negroes, and in that year there were 392 deaths from Asiatic Cholera, which pressed particularly on that class.

As my desire is to base all my reasonings and conclusions on *facts*, I shall here present an abstract of the Register's report which I have made out with much care, so that the reader will be able to judge for himself of the legitimacy of my deductions. The original table embraces all the deaths, and causes of death in the city of Charleston for 18 years, viz: from 1828 to 1845, both included, and in making my abstract, I have divided this term of years into three periods, of six years; and as I have wished to present the facts in a form which would allow of comparison with other places, I have in the main, adopted the plan of Mr. Farr, the distinguished statistician of England. I have also found a valuable guide, as well as a mine of interesting facts in the able report of Mr. Shattuck, on the Census of Boston, for 1845.

The causes as will be seen in the table, are divided into—1st. Zimotic Diseases; 2d. Sporadic Diseases; 3d. Old Age and external causes, such as violence, drowning, poisoning, &c.

Zimotic, is a term used by Mr. Farr to designate all epidemic, endemic and contagious diseases. It is the property of Zimotic diseases, to prevail more at one season than at another, or more in one locality than another, and to become Epidemic, Endemic, or contagious under certain circumstances. This class, as will be seen, includes all fevers arising from morbid poisons, as, intermittents, remittents, yellow, and typhus fevers; also small-pox, measles, scarlatina, influenza, &c., and the greater or less number of deaths from this class has been assumed as the best test of the salubrity of a climate.

Sporadic Diseases embrace all those which do not belong to the above class, as our table will show.

Old age, and external causes, cannot be called diseases, and should, therefore, (particularly the latter,) be separated from the other classes in estimating the influence of climate on health.

The following table as I have stated, extends over eighteen years, which are divided into three periods of six years each. The aggregate number of deaths for each period, is given from all causes; the number from each specified cause; and the percentage which each one bears to the whole, &c.

TABLE. B.
Abstract of the Causes of Death in Charleston, from 1828, *to* 1845.

CAUSES OF DEATH.	1828 to 1833	1834 to 1839	1840 to 1845	1828 to 1833	1834 to 1839	1840 to 1845
All Causes,	4143	5229	3583			
Specified Causes,	3968	5080	3503			
1. Zimotic Diseases,	952	1900	765	23,99	37,40	21,83
SPORADIC DISEASES.						
2. Of uncertain or general seat,	506	548	426	12,75	10,78	12,16
3. Of the Nervous System,	593	605	606	14,94	11,90	17,29
4. Of the organs of Respiration,	910	878	813	22,93	17,28	23,20
5. Organs of Circulation,	16	27	33	0,40	0,53	0,94
6. Organs of Digestion,	417	549	399	10,50	10,80	11,39
7. Urinary Organs,	6	2	5	0,15	0,05	0,14
8. Organs of Generation,	35	51	48	0,88	1,00	1,37
9. Organs of Locomotion,	21	14	14	0,56	0,27	0,39
10. Integumentary System,	7	9	7	0,17	0,17	0,19
11. Old Age,	311	299	226	7,83	5,88	6,45
12. Deaths from External causes,	194	198	161	4,88	3,89	4,59

No. of Deaths in the Periods. — In each 100 there were in

Longevity in reference to Life Insurance.

[TABLE B. CONTINUED.]

CAUSES OF DEATH.	No. of Deaths in the periods, 1828 to 1833	1834 to 1839	1840 to 1845	In each 100 there were in 1828 to 1833	1834 to 1839	1840 to 1845
Class 1st.						
Cholera,	14	19	4	,35	0,37	0,11
Cholera Infantum,	5	63	71	,12	1,23	·2,02
Cholera, Asiatic	0	392	0	,00	7,70	,00
Croup,	43	39	43	1,08	,76	1,22
Diarrhœa,	104	66	25	2,62	1,29	,71
Dysentery,	45	77	51	2,62	1,29	,71
Bowel Complaint,	83	23	5	2,09	,45	,14
Erysipelas,	4	2	2	,10	,03	,05
Fever,	43	110	44	1,08	2,16	1,23
" Inflammatory,	4	8	2	,10	,15	,05
" Intermittent,	3	5	24	,07	,09	,68
" Remittent,	93	144	50	2,34	2,83	1,42
" Country,	78	35	11	1,96	,68	,31
" Yellow,	58	562	26	1,46	11,06	,74
" Congestive,	0	4	12	,00	,07	,34
" Typhus,	49	79	93	1,23	1,55	2,65
Hooping Cough,	106	70	61	2,66	1,37	1,74
Influenza,	11	18	10	,27	,35	,28
Measles,	26	43	31	,65	,84	,88
Scarlatina and Sorethroat,	78	127	127	1,96	2,50	3,62
Small Pox,	63	0	53	1,58	,00	1,51
Syphilis,	1	0	2	,02	,00	,05
Thrush,	23	13	18	0,57	,25	,51
Parotitis,	0	1	0	,00	,01	,00
Dengue,	18	0	0	,45	,00	,00
Class 2d.						
Abscess,	14	16	13	,85	,35	,37
Atrophy.	1	1	14	,02	,01	,39
Cancer,	26	15	30	,65	,29	,85
Debility,	128	125	70	3,22	2,45	1,90
Dropsy,	285	328	243	7,18	6,45	6,93
Gout,	4	1	1	,10	,01	,02
Hæmorrhage,	5	14	10	,12	,27	,28
Inflammation,	5	5	0	,12	,09	,00
Mortification,	10	4	3	,25	,07	,08
Scrofula,	12	20	12	,30	,39	,34
Tumor,	4	3	0	,10	,05	,00
Marasmus,	11	15	27	,27	,29	,77
Spine Diseases,	1	1	3	,02	,01	,08
Class 3d.						
Apoplexy,	98	111	113	2,46	2,18	3,22
Cephalitis,	31	57	38	,78	1.12	1,08
Convulsions,	189	154	138	4,76	3,03	3,93
Delirium Tremens,	5	27	3	,12	,53	,08

[TABLE B. CONTINUED.]

| | No. of Deaths in the periods. ||| In each 100 there were in |||
CAUSES OF DEATH.	1828 to 1833	1834 to 1839	1840 to 1845	1828 to 1833	1834 to 1839	1840 to 1845
Coup de Soleil,	3	1	1	,07	,01	,02
Epilepsy,	51	27	13	1,27	,53	,37
Hydrocephalus,	17	29	17	,42	,57	,48
Insanity,	17	16	18	,42	,35	,51
Paralysis,	57	60	54	1,43	1,18	1,54
Tetanus,	7	18	29	,17	,35	,82
Trismus Nascentium,	90	83	160	2,31	1,63	4,56
Cramp,	8	0	0	,20	,00	,00
Nervous Affections,	5	5	0	,12	,09	,00
Brain, Diseases of	15	17	22	,37	,33	,62

CLASS 4TH.

Asthma,	28	24	31	,70	,47	,88
Consumption,	665	565	561	16,75	11,12	16,01
Hydrothorax,	70	88	70	1,76	1,73	1,99
Laryngitis,	2	0	2	,05	,00	,05
Bronchitis,	3	9	8	,07	,17	,22
Pleurisy,	33	23	17	,83	,45	,48
Pneumonia,	5	5	17	,12	,09	,48
Inflammation of Lungs,	12	29	21	,30	,57	,59
Hæmmorhage of Lungs,	1	3	0	,02	,05	,00
Lungs, Diseases of	10	6	8	,25	,12	,22
Catarrhal Fever and Catarrah,	81	126	78	2,04	2,48	2,22

CLASS 5TH.

Aneurism,	1	4	3	,02	,07	,08
Heart, Diseases of	15	23	30	,37	,45	,85

CLASS 6TH.

Colic,	32	28	14	,80	,55	,39
Dyspepsia,	3	3	5	,07	,05	,14
Enteritis, Gastritis, Inflammation of Bowels,	60	99	90	1,51	1,94	2,56
Hernia,	4	3	7	,10	,05	,09
Intussusception,	1	1	0	,02	,02	,00
Peritonitis,	1	8	2	,02	,10	,05
Teething,	160	253	181	4,03	4,97	5,16
Worms, and Worm Fever,	81	76	40	2,04	1,49	1,13
Liver, Diseases of	2	1	0	,05	,01	,00
Jaundice,	12	11	11	,30	,21	,31
Organs, Diseases of	2	4	10	,05	,07	,28

CLASS 7TH.

Diabetes,	00	00	00	,00	,00	,00
Cystitis,	00	1	2	,00	,01	,05
Gravel,	5	1	2	,12	,01	,05
Nephritis,	1	0	1	,02	,00	,02

Longevity in reference to Life Insurance.

[TABLE B. CONTINUED.]

	No. of Deaths in the periods.			In each 100 there were in		
CAUSES OF DEATH.	1828 to 1833	1834 to 1839	1840 to 1845	1828 to 1833	1834 to 1839	1840 to 1845
CLASS 8TH.						
Childbirth,	29	38	34			
Puerperal Fever,	2	5	2	,05	,09	,05
Organs, Diseases of	4	8	12	,10	,10	,34
CLASS 9TH.						
Rheumatism,	21	11	14	,52	,21	,39
Joints, Diseases of	0	3	0	,00	,05	,00
CLASS 10TH.						
Fistula,	0	1	0	,00	,01	,00
Ulcer,	3	3	2	,07	,05	,05
Skin, Diseases of	4	5	5	,10	,09	,14
CLASS 11TH.						
Old Age,	311	299	226	7,83	5,88	6,45
CLASS 12TH.						
Burns and Scalds,	8	3	5			
Casualties,	40	55	48			
Drinking Cold Water,	0	0	0			
Intemperance,	93	80	45			
Drowned,	26	36	43			
Executed,	0	1	2			
Fractures,	2	5	1			
Cold, Effects of	13	7	1			
Hydrophobia,	2	0	1			
Murdered,	0	0	1			
Poisoned,	2	1	2			
Suffocated,	0	4	2			
Suicide,	8	6	10			
CLASS 13TH.						
Causes not Specified,	175	149	90			

The reader cannot fail to be struck, on the first glance at this table, by the great disparity exhibited in the gross mortality of the three periods; and the fact is equally prominent, that this disparity is attributable to the increase or decrease of *Zimotic* diseases. The mortality for each of the periods was as follows: 4143—5229—3583. From the *Zimotic* class the deaths were in each period; 952—1900—765, or for each 100, a percentage of 23,99—37,40—21,83. Here is strong evidence of the influence of endemics and epidemics over mortality; and the general fact has been taken as sufficient proof of the insalubrity of Charleston, and other cities similarly situated as to climate. The average mortality for a series of years, has been estimated by Dr. Dunglison in his work on "*Human Health*," at 1 in 36, which places this city below, and very far below most of the northern cities of the United States.

The important question now comes up, viz: who are they that die from these Zimotic diseases? Are they acclimated citizens of Charleston, or are they not? and I beg the reader to bear in mind the general remarks which have been made on the subject of *acclimation*. The deaths in the second period of our table exceeded those of the third by 1135 or 148 per cent. By turning to class 1st. in table B, it will be seen that the deaths from yellow fever in three periods were 58—562—26, a very striking contrast certainly. Look at the heads fever, bilious fever, &c., and we find a greater mortality from these causes, also in the second, than in either of the other periods; many of which deaths, no doubt, were erroneously excluded from the head, yellow fever.

The table C, which we give below, besides some other interesting facts, reveals the following one which will go far towards answering the question, who are they that die from the endemic diseases of the climate? viz: the deaths for the "*not natives*," were in each of the three periods, 764—1418—659, showing that the mortality amongst this class of population rises and falls as these causes act with greater or less force. If the table be taken in detail, year by year, this law is seen to be invariable. In the great epidemic of 1838 for example, there were 482 deaths amongst the *non-natives*, and so on with the other years. A portion of the deaths from yellow fever, are amongst native children of the city, who, as we have stated, though far less liable to this disease than foreigners, are not considered as fully acclimated. It should be remembered also, that 392 of the deaths, (or 8 per cent) of the second period, were from Asiatic cholera, which should be excluded from the calculation in estimating the influence of climate on the acclimated.

The table on which our calculations have been based, as before stated, is for the eighteen years, commencing at 1828, and ending 1st. January, 1846, but it will be seen that the following table extends back to 1822. The early years are wanting in some of the details, but they are still of sufficient value to merit a place with the others, and can be easily separated.

TABLE C.

Showing the gross Mortality for each year, and the ratio of the Whites, Blacks, Natives, Non-natives, Sexes, &c.

	WHITES Male.	WHITES Fem's.	COLORED Male.	COLORED Fem's.	TOTAL WHIT'S	TOTAL BLCK'S	GRAND TOTAL	NOT NAT'VE	NAT'VE	DEATHS OF WHITES.	DEATHS OF BLACKS.	
1822	284	142	253	246	426	499	925	—	629	—	—	
1823	217	132	213	250	349	463	812	185	677	—	—	
1824	434	198	222	205	632	427	1059	382	675	—	—	
1825	228	125	253	234	353	487	840	165	—	—	—	
1826	203	108	217	236	311	453	764	—	—	—	—	236 deaths fm. yel. fever.
1827	258	124	216	205	382	421	803	—	—	—	—	
1828	232	126	222	213	358	435	793	168	625	One in 36,14	One in 39,91	63 "
1829	183	124	205	250	307	455	762	102	660	" 42,28	" 38,15	26 "
1830	209	120	199	235	329	434	763	143	620	" 39,45	" 40,00	—
1831	164	114	218	237	278	455	733	150	583	" 46,69	" 37,93	32 "
1832	142	108	161	119	250	310	560	96	464	" 51,91	" 55,35	—
1833	145	91	136	170	236	306	542	105	437	" 55,00	" 55,75	—
1834	192	116	158	226	308	384	692	166	526	" 42,14	" 44,16	49 "
1835	189	112	176	187	301	363	664	181	483	" 43,12	" 46,44	26 "
1836	196	123	443	410	319	853	1172	181	991	" 40,68	" 19,61	392 "	Asiatic Chol.
1837	172	102	180	176	274	356	630	144	456	" 47,37	" 46,79	—
1838	551	158	277	223	709	500	1209	482	727	" 18,30	" 33,00	354 "	yellow fever.
1839	307	127	195	227	434	422	856	264	592	" 29,93	" 39,00	134 "
1840	184	73	177	171	257	348	605	179	426	" 50,70	" 46,64	23 "
1841	120	80	187	173	200	360	560	94	456	" 65,15	" 44,80	—
1842	171	88	165	170	259	335	594	113	481	" 50,30	" 47,85	—
1843	131	83	237	246	214	483	697	89	608	" 60,88	" 32,98	2 "
1844	109	79	173	192	188	365	553	108	445	" 69,30	" 43,36	1 "
1845	119	127	153	171	246	324	570	76	494	" 52,96	" 48,54	—

Many of the causes of death which by the arbitrary arrangement of Mr. Farr are thrown into class second, are but sequilæ of fevers, and really belong to the first or Zimotic class.

Debility, for example, (which is but another name for obscure organic lesions,) caused in the periods respectively 128—125—70. So with *dropsy*, which is here a *symptom* of some visceral obstruction following fever. The deaths from this cause were, 285---328---243. A reference to table B, will show that the greatest mortality from *debility* and *dropsy* was in those periods when fevers prevailed most, and consequently pressed more upon the unacclimated, than upon the acclimated. I do not wish to be understood as attributing all of our dropsies to this source, but certainly a large portion of those in miasmatic regions are the consequences of fevers.

The table of mortality shows a number of deaths, from what in Charleston, is called *country fever*, and which affords a very instructive illustration of what may be termed *local climates*. If one of the native or acclimated inhabitants of the city, during the sickly season, goes out into the surrounding country and sleeps a night, he is almost certain to be attacked with a malignant form of marsh fever, which is more fatal than yellow fever. The inhabitants are very cautious in avoiding such exposure, and in estimating the influence of the climate of the city on the acclimated, these cases should be left out. Mobile and New-Orleans are not similarly situated in this particular; their suburbs and the surrounding country, are comparatively healthy, though they are not free in all parts from intermittents and remittents.

The same reasoning applies to our sixth class, or diseases of the *digestive organs*. The number of deaths from this class, were in the three periods, 417---549---399; the greatest mortality corresponding with the prevalence of fevers, or that class of diseases which affect the unacclimated most.

The deaths from *old age*, (which is rather a vague term as used in bills of mortality,) were in the periods, 311---299---226; the lowest mortality being in the period most exempt from fevers. Many of these cases no doubt were premature deaths from the influence of malaria many years back, before there was a well marked *city climate*, and when the inhabitants were subject to intermittent and bilious fevers. The older the town (in this country,) the greater of course will be the number of the acclimated, if not disturbed by emigration.

Typhus, as is well known, is not a disease of the South; the deaths for the three periods in Charleston from this cause were, 49---79---93; or 1,23,---1,55, and 2,65 per cent on the whole deaths of the periods. As I have before remarked, I have not met a well marked case since I have been in Mobile. This disease, in the towns of Great Britain, is one of the great outlets of life.

The tables we have given, afford much material for reflexion, but our space bids us hurry on. *Fever* has been looked on as the great outlet at the South, and many of our readers will no doubt be surprised to learn that the deaths in Charleston for the last 18 years, from all malarial fevers (excluding yellow fever,) viz: fever, bilious, intermittent, country, congestive and remittent fevers, have been but 656, and that during this time, there has been no epidemic; the highest number of deaths from all, in any one year, having been but 81. I have no doubt as before stated, that many of these cases, in yellow fever years, were from the latter disease, as cases of yellow fever which do not present, what by some is regarded as the characteristic symptom *black vomit* are often put down by the physician as bilious fever, to avoid remarks. Such a result in a city so far south, with apparently such an unfavorable topography, and with a population varying during the whole time but little from 30,000 could not have been anticipated. Many of these fevers too, do not properly belong to the city, but have been contracted by sleeping imprudently in the country, and on hunting and fishing parties, &c. Suppose the population of Charleston eighteen years ago, had been scattered over the *bilious fever* districts of the South, how different would have been the result? Who can estimate within 1,000, the mortality which these diseases would have produced?

The aggregate of deaths from yellow fever during the periods, varied but little from the above; it was 646, and this is a disease which we have shown, affects almost exclusively the unacclimated. In estimating fairly, therefore, the climate of the city proper, we should exclude yellow fever, country fever, and a considerable portion of other miasmatic fevers.

An examination of our table shows, that although there were light *endemic* visitations, there have really been no *epidemics* of yellow fever for the last twenty years, except those of 1838 and 1839, and in these two years the disease was brought into action by extraordinary causes. A medical friend of Charleston, who is familiar with the facts, and of high authority writes me, "during this year (1838,) in April, a large part of the city was destroyed by fire, leaving an immense surface covered with decomposable matter, exposed to the rays of the sun; *many of the cellars and sinks were filled with water which it was impossible to remove, and in this very situation, there was a vast number of foreigners occupied in removing the ruins.*" When there is an increased demand for mechanics and laborers, they will of course come in from other places, and we thus have not only a cause assigned for the disease, but the subjects supplied for it to feed on. The same causes were still in operation to some extent in the following year 1839. The deaths of *non-natives* in these years were, 482, and 262, more than double the mortality in ordinary years amongst this class.

I have been disappointed in my endeavors to get recent statistics from New-York and Philadelphia. There are some very able articles by Dr. G. Emerson, in the Amer. Journ. of Med. Sci., on the Vital Statistics of the latter, down as late as 1830. The mortality was in Philadelphia according to Dr E., as below.

Philadelphia,	1827 to 1830, from	Zimotic class, (average)		25,17 pr. ct.
England,	1838 to 1842,	" " " "		19 to 21 "
Philadelphia,	1820 to 1830,	" fevers alone "		13,5 "
"	1820 to 1830,	" bowel complaints "		11,5 "
"	" " "	consumption "		14,7 "

In Charleston the average for eighteen years for bowel complaints, was but 5 per cent; and for fevers, including the two epidemics of yellow fever in the second period of table B, was, 11,41 or 2 per cent less than Philadelphia; for the other two periods embracing the twelve years, the average was under 8 per cent. It would seem from these facts, that the mortality from *fevers* is much greater in Philadelphia than Charleston. Charleston of late years, has been becoming more healthy; I do not know how it is in Philadelphia.

Dr. Emerson has shown that the mortality from fevers in Philadelphia, was principally in the "outskirts and environs" of the city, and this is strikingly the case with the intermittents and remittents of Charleston, Mobile and New-Orleans. Paving would seem to be the most efficient means of expelling these fevers from cities.

I must now bring to a close these brief remarks on the Zimotic class, and refer the reader to the tables given, which will tell their own tale to those familiar with vital statistics. It will be seen that Charleston will compare with any city in the Union, as regards cholera, dysentery, diarrhœa, bowel complaints, &c., and we shall show in its proper place, the great advantage Charleston enjoys in immunity from these disorders in early life. When we reflect on the facts given, and the comparative immunity which Charleston (as well as other southern towns,) enjoys from the other scourges of the Zimotic class, viz; small-pox, measles in severe form, scarlatina, hooping cough, and typhus, (from all of which combined, I have not in my practice seen more than from 15 to 20 deaths in the last eleven years in Mobile,) we may fairly conclude that the climate of southern seaports is not so very bad after all.

I will now make a few cursory remarks on some of the other classes.

Of class 3d. or nervous system, I shall notice but a single disease, viz; *trismus nascentium*, the deaths from which, in the three periods were, 90—83—160; or 2,31—1,63 and 4,56 per cent on the whole deaths of the periods. This disease is well known to increase as the tropic is approached, and I presume that it is in Charleston as elsewhere, confined mostly to the *black* children.

Class 4th. or Diseases of the Organs of Respiration, forms a very interesting point of comparison between northern and southern climates. Though the mortality from the *whole* class, is, I believe, generally admitted to be greater at the North than at the South; yet it must be confessed, that modern statistics have rendered it doubtful whether the same rule applies to tubercular consumption alone; even in the West Indies this disease is found to prevail to a considerable extent. In Charleston, the deaths from *all* diseases of the organs of respiration, were for the three periods, 910—878—813, being 22,93—17,28, and 23,30 per cent on all the deaths. It is apparent, that though the *percentage* of deaths from this cause, fluctuated between 17 and 23 per cent, still there was great uniformity in the actual number of deaths for the periods, as well as the ratio to the living population. Whenever the deaths from the Zimotic class swelled the bills of mortality, the relative proportion of the other classes would, of course, be diminished, thus affording conclusive evidence of the fallacy of estimating the force of causes of mortality in this way alone. The greatest percentage of deaths from diseases of the respiratory organs, is seen in the healthiest period, viz; 23,20 per cent.

It would appear from the statistics we have given, that the mortality from the 4th. class in Charleston, is really great; the *whole* mortality for the last period, (from 1840 to 1845,) being one death to 51,12, of the living, and the deaths for this period (which was the most healthy,) being 23,20 per cent for class 4th. In all England the deaths from this class from 1838 to 1842, fluctuated but a fraction from 27 per cent, and in Boston, there was a steady decrease of deaths from this class, from 32,70 down to 23,97 per cent from 1811 to the year 1845. The deaths in Charleston from *consumption* alone were for the three periods 665—565, and 561, or 16,75—11,12—16,01 per cent on all the deaths. In Boston they were for the four periods of Mr. Shattuck's table 25,14—21,50—15,30, and 15,13 per cent, showing a constant *decrease*, while the Zimotic class during the same period, exhibits a corresponding *increase*, viz; 15,85—21,32—27,56, and 28,36 per cent. It may, I think, be taken as a fixed rule that as one rises the other falls, and that consequently the percentage of deaths from one class alone, affords very unsatisfactory information. I should have remarked that the deaths from all acute diseases of the lungs in Charleston, give an aggregate for eighteen years of but 182 deaths, or an average of ten a year in a population of about 30,000.

The statistics, however, of both Boston and Charleston, I think are very unsatisfactory as to the agency of their respective climates in producing tubercular consumption. 1st. Because many who have *"weak lungs,"* or actual phthisis, leave Boston, and come to Charleston and other southern countries to die, in the vain hope of cure from change of climate. 2d. Because the negroes, who are very subject in towns to phthisis, cannot be separated in the report of the Register from the whites; nor can we separate the deaths of foreigners from those of the natives in this or any other specified disease. These causes must of course greatly confuse our statistics. Another remark of considerable weight I think, is this; that a rapid influx of population into a northern city, will produce a very opposite influence on the general mortality, as well as the mortality from specified causes; no one will deny, for example, that an influx of foreigners into Charleston, will greatly swell the bills of mortality, and particularly the list of deaths from *fevers.* In Boston an influx increases the mortality from Zimotic diseases of a different kind, and the proportion of diseases of the lungs diminish in a corresponding ratio.

The census of Boston shows the following rapid increase of population.

1830,	–	61,392
1835,	–	78,603
1840,	–	85,000
1845,	–	114,366

From the great prosperity of this city, there has been a demand for the active, productive class of population, and we consequently see a great influx of the young, vigorous and enterprising. The census of this city, taken in 1845, shows the extraordinary fact, of a population 36 per cent. of whom are between the ages of 20 and 35! In Charleston, the heavy mortality would fall upon this class, whereas in Boston its influence is to *decrease* the ratio of mortality, and if I am not mistaken, in diseases of the lungs particularly, taking a population of this kind in the aggregate, does a table of mortality show the influence of climate? One of the strong characteristics of consumption is, that it becomes hereditary, and here we see a sturdy, young population coming in and disturbing the natural course of things, so as to upset all calculations about the influence of climate. The greatest mortality in Boston, as we shall see, is in childhood, the deaths under five years being nearly 47 per cent. I may be mistaken, but it really seems to me, that in view of the above considerations, one death in forty-six or forty-eight of the living in the city of Boston, is by no means an indication of a low ratio of mortality; the climate on the natives alone, would probably tell a different tale. But my object in this investigation is truth, and I shall be happy to be corrected; it is of no consequence to me which has the best climate for health, Charleston or Boston. Our Yankee friends certainly have the "go-a-head" principle in the highest degree.

Class 6th. or Diseases of the Digestive organs is also an important one, as it is considered one of the main outlets of life, in southern climates, but we must deal with it briefly. The deaths from these causes were 417—549 and 399 for the three periods, or 10,50—10,80 and 11,39 per cent of all the deaths. The greatest number, as before stated, is seen in the middle period when fevers prevailed most, and the unacclimated consequently have swollen the per centage of this class. In Boston, the percentage from this class was 6,75—8,20 and 9,50, from 1821 to 1845, and I think we may fairly conclude the per centage is not greater amongst the *acclimated* of Charleston.

From 1838 to 1842, the bills for *all* England, show a fluctuation in this class from 5,89 to 6,64 per cent. I have not at hand details for the *cities* of England, but they probably will show as high mortality in this class, as Charleston. I will detain the reader on but one more point of this class and the facts will probably surprise most northern readers.

Diseases of the *liver* and *spleen* have been looked upon as the great curses of southern latitudes. The deaths from *all* affections of the liver, for the three periods were 59—62 and 39, being but 1,48—1,22 and 1,11 per cent on all the deaths, and but three deaths in eighteen years from diseases of the spleen. Persons at the North, who have read Johnson on the Liver, and other works of English writers on diseases of *hot climates*, have often, without sufficient investigation, regarded the Southern States as similarly situated; but here we see that in Charleston (and so with Mobile and New-Orleans,) diseases of the liver are almost unknown, while in Bengal we are told. "one half the deaths are from diseases of the liver." I can declare with confidence, and my professional brethren here will sustain me, that I see fewer diseases of the liver in Mobile, than of any important organ in the body. I do not think I exaggerate, when I say, that the cases in my practice, belonging to Mobile, do not exceed one a year. This remark only applies to the southern seaports. I have no apology to offer for the bilious fever regions of the interior of the Southern States, where all malarial disorders are seen in abundance.

On class 7th, Diseases of the Urinary Organs—I will remark that diabetes is extremely rare, as are calculous diseases. All the cases of Stone I have operated on, have been from the interior or from other States.

Mortality of the Negroes.—The Statistics of Charleston, afford some very curious and instructive information on this point—the influences of climate and social condition, are both strongly illustrated here. The fact must be admitted, from the bills of Mortality, that the deaths amongst this class are double in Philadelphia, and treble in Boston, over those of Charleston, however we may differ as to the causes operating to produce such a result. I brought forward numerous facts on a former occasion to show that this mortality was mainly attributable to the influence of cold on a race of beings who were created and intended for tropical climates, and my opinion has remained unchanged, though I have no doubt that the social condition of the negro at the North, will account for a very large per centage, possibly half of this mortality. The negro by nature is indolent and improvident in all climates, and there can be no question, that many die in the Northern cities, because they have neglected to provide those comforts which are necessary to protect them against cold. The following tables of mortality amongst the blacks will speak for themselves.

Deaths of Blacks in Charleston.

1830, one in 40,00,		
1831, " " 37,93,	1841, one in 44.80	
1832, " " 55,95,	1842, " " 47,85	
1833, " " 55,75,	1843, " " 32,98	
1834, " " 44,16,	1844, " " 43,36	
1835, " " 66,44,	1845, " " 48,54	
1836, cholera 19,64,		
1837 one in 46,79,		
1838, " " 33,00,		
1839, " " 39,00,		
1840, " " 46,64,		

PHILADELPHIA.

1821, one in 16,9
1822, " " 21,5
1823, " " 17,5
1824, " " 17,5
1825, " " 27,0
1826, " " 26,1
1827, " " 18,9
1828, " " 20,8
1829, " " 23,7
1830, " " 27,2

Thus the average for 16 years, (excluding the Cholera year,) in Charleston, shows a mortality in the colored population, of one in 44—while in Philadelphia, the average for 10 years is one in 21,7. I have not been able as yet to procure tables of mortality from Boston, New York, and Baltimore, but the mortality amongst the free blacks of these cities, I have seen put down by competent authorities at one in 15, one in 18, and one in 32. We have the authority of Dr. Niles, for putting the mortality of the free colored in Baltimore, at one in 32, while *the slaves give the proportion of one in 77*. There can be no question that if the free colored in Charleston, were separated from the slaves, a still less mortality than one in 44 would be exhibited. No where in the reach of history, though we can trace them back at least 2000 years before the Christian Era, have the negroes shown themselves capable of supplying their physical, to say nothing of moral wants—they are every where when left alone, indolent and improvident, and consequently subject to greater mortality, than they should be. There is a large proportion of *mulattoes* in Charleston, which should be taken into consideration when estimating the influence of climate and social condition on the colored class,—for I have given reasons on a former occasion for the opinion that they are a degenerate *Hybrid Race*, and subject to much greater mortality and lower average duration of life than either whites or blacks.

Though a native of the South, I am not conscious of being influenced in the opinions I am expressing by prejudices of education, and certainly not by personal interest, and am not one of those who regard slavery as a great blessing, even to the Southern States. Though I am entirely free from any scruples of conscience, as to the present condition of the blacks in these States, I should have no objection to see them all shipped back to the torrid Zone, if it could be done with humanity to the blacks, and a due regard to the constitutional rights of their owners. Such a course now, would be greatly prejudicial to the happiness of the slave, and to the wealth both of the master and of these States. But the future is always pregnant with great events, which no wisdom can foresee—on the one hand, the the black population is accumulating with such fearful rapidity on the Gulf States, that grave questions must be debated ere long as to their future destination. On the other hand, when we look at the mighty social movements in progress all over the world, it is not unreasonable to suppose, that a substitute for this labor at the South, may be found. Should a more liberal policy prevail in China, a few of her starving millions might be spared, to cultivate our Rice and Cotton lands, even cheaper than by slave labor.

The negroes of the South, I am satisfied, from long personal observation, not only in the different portions of the United States, but also in Great Britain and France, are the happiest population on the face of the globe. They never yet from the building of the Pyramids of Egypt, (on which they worked as slaves) to the present day, under any circumstances in which they have been placed, have been able to conceive those delicious abstract notions of liberty, which we are told, make the bosom of the half starved operative, swell with pride and exultation. Liberty is a want which they are incapable of enjoying, and do not feel —they have no care about the temporal wants of the future, and are less disturbed by wants, both moral and physical, than the nobility of England.

To those who believe that the excessive mortality amongst this class at the North, is attributable to climate alone, and who believe that the condition of the negro is capable of being improved by emancipation; I will say, without fear of contradiction, that if health and longevity (and I might add happy faces,) are evidences of physical comfort and content, they are in a better condition in Charleston, (and the Southern States generally,) than any laboring class on the face of the globe. It is a remarkable fact that this class in Charleston, shows not only a lower mortality than any laboring class of any country, but a lower mortality than the aggregate population (including the higher classes, nobility and all,) of any country in Europe, except England, with which it is about on a par. If we could separate the free colored, the ratio would doubtless be below England, as it is now below her towns taken apart from the country. Freedom and climate combined in Boston, are far more destructive to the negro than slavery and Asiatic Cholera at the South. This scourge, which in 1836 in Charleston fell most heavily upon the negroes, raised the mortality for that year, to one in 20; while in Boston, it *averages* about 1 in 15.

The Ages at Death, of a population, have been regarded as amongst the most essential facts for determining its longevity, compared with other places. It is necessary however, to make such comparisons, that the census should be taken frequently, in order that the dying in each period of life, may be compared with the living of the same ages. Otherwise we cannot compare one population with itself, at different epochs, or with another. These and many other details which are required, are deficient in the Charleston tables. I have the ages of the dead and the months, in which they died, only for the last 6 years of our table B., viz: from 1840 to 1846, and I will here give an abstract of these years, which will be useful to us in elucidating the remainder of our remarks. During these 6 years, there was no epidemic of yellow fever, and I think the facts not unsatisfactory as illustrative of the influence of the climate of Charleston, upon its acclimated citizens, though like every other place, it may be visited by occasional seasons, when a somewhat greater mortality will be seen.

It should be remarked also, that I am unable from the Charleston tables in my possession, to separate the blacks and whites in the table below—this is much to be regretted, as the longevity of each class cannot be got at without the ages and other full details.

TABLE D.

Of Mortality for Charleston, from 1840 to 1846, (six years,) showing the Mortality of the different Months, and the Ages at Death.

	Under 1 year	1 to 5	5 to 10	10 to 20	20 to 30	30 to 40	40 to 50	50 to 60	60 to 70	70 to 80	80 to 90	90 to 100	100 to 110	110 to 120	Total.	Aver. age.
January,	35	33	9	11	23	22	28	18	17	16	15	6	3	0	236	39,33
February,	29	28	16	13	29	30	31	17	15	17	7	2	0	0	233	38,63
March,	37	28	12	14	28	32	27	22	26	16	5	3	0	0	253	42,16
April,	52	34	13	23	28	37	40	30	24	22	9	4	1	1	318	53,00
May,	67	40	17	33	33	22	30	18	22	17	8	3	0	1	311	51,83
June,	74	46	17	24	33	32	25	29	22	11	10	3	0	0	326	54,33
July,	86	53	16	24	46	32	27	19	22	13	9	0	0	0	349	58,16
August,	85	70	21	22	39	43	30	21	18	10	6	2	1	0	373	62,16
September,	57	44	11	24	62	40	35	32	23	16	8	7	0	1	373	62,16
October,	40	40	4	14	32	36	37	21	17	13	12	6	1	0	271	45,16
November,	53	34	3	20	29	32	27	16	18	21	7	2	0	0	250	41,66
December,	44	33	11	18	38	49	35	21	7	13	16	3	3	0	292	48,66
Total, -	659	483	150	239	420	395	372	262	231	185	112	46	12	3	3569	594,83
Average, -	109,83	80,50	25,00	39,83	70,00	65,83	62,00	43,66	38,50	30,83	18,66	7,66	2,00	,50		
Per centage,	18,46	13,53	4,20	6,69	11,76	11,07	10,42	7,34	6,44	5,18	3,13	1,28	,33	,08		
	31,99															

For the purpose of ascertaining the comparative longevity of different places, various methods have been adopted, and tables constructed—none of these are perhaps free from objections, but when all are taken together, their various relations considered, and due allowance being made for local and temporary circumstances, they afford valuable information. We have no space, and are wanting in data, for making a full investigation of this part of our subject—we will merely give a few facts, and tables, after the plan of Mr. Shattuck, by which others, if so disposed, may make comparisons with other places.

"There are various modes, says Mr. Shattuck, by which the element of the ages at death, has been applied to measure the average health of a people." He enumerates five, which I shall follow in his order.

FIRST METHOD.—*By ascertaining the proportion of all the deaths that occur at specific periods of life.*—The subjoined table, will illustrate this method, and it will be seen that it is taken for Charleston, from the preceding table :

In each 100, there were in

	Charleston.	Boston.	New-York
Under 5	31,99	46,62	50,00
5 to 10	4,20	4,46	
10 to 20	6,69	5,29	
20 to 30	11,76	11,71	
30 to 40	11,07	10,12	
40 to 50	10,42	6,97	
50 to 60	7,34	4,88	
60 to 70	6,44	4,18	
70 to 80	5,18	3,69	
80 to 90	3,13	1,79	
90 to 100	1,28	,29	

These estimates are based on six years for Charleston, viz; 1840 to 1845; and for Boston five years, from 1841 to 1845; and show the proportion per cent of deaths at the ages specified in the first column. Although this table does little towards settling the question of longevity, it affords valuable information of a different kind. In the tables given by Mr. Shattuck in his report on the census of Boston, taken in 1845, it appears that the per centage of mortality amongst children under five years, increased steadily during the previous thirty-five years, from 33,64 to 46,62 per cent, and when we recollect that the mortality in Boston during the last five years was one in forty-seven, it shows that this period of life is very heavily pressed upon, in that city. In Charleston, the average mortality for the last six years, including whites and blacks, was one in fifty-one, while the mortality under five years of age, was but 31,99 per cent, and was of course, much lower in those periods when the mortality was great from *fevers*.

I have not extended the comparison of mortality in early life, with other cities, but the mortality amongst children in all the large towns, North of the Potomac, is greatly above that of Charleston. Children in those cities, suffer much more from the diseases of summer, as well as the Zimotic and inflammatory diseases of winter.

In the large *towns* of England, 38 per cent die *within the first year*, and in Charleston, 15 per cent, and in the country districts of England, 22 per cent.

SECOND METHOD. *By ascertaining the proportion that survived specific ages, of all that die.* The table below, exhibits the number that died, but survived specific ages, and is deduced from the last table; the results of calculations in several other places, are added for comparisons; for Charleston it includes all colors.

	CHARLESTON.	BOSTON.	PRESTON IN ENGLAND.	NEWTON.
At birth,	100.00	100.00	100.00	100.00
Surviving 5 years,	68.01	53.38	82.40	81.00
" 10 "	63.81	48.92	81.10	76.75
" 20 "	57.12	43.63	76.30	70.50
" 30 "	45.36	31.92	72.30	63.75
" 40 "	34.30	21.80	63.40	56.25
" 50 "	23.88	14.83	56.00	48.00
" 60 "	16.54	9.95	45.10	38.75
" 70 "	10.10	5.77	25.40	29.00
" 80 "	4.92	2.08	8.00	14.25
" 90 "	1.79	.29	1.30	3.75

This table shows, that in Charleston of 100 children born, 68 survived the 5th year; 34 the 40th year; 10 the 70th year, &c. If a large number die under five years, the per centage of all above, will be less, and so with the succeeding ages. Mr. Shattuck gives some instructive facts, to show how mortality presses upon certain ages and classes. In the Catholic burying ground in Boston, (the poor laboring class) 61.39 per cent of the deaths, were under 5 years, and but 5½ per cent lived to see 50 years, and 2 per cent, 70 ; average duration of life, 13.

The two foregoing tables, though teaching important facts, are by no means conclusive as to the longevity of a population. As much depends upon the character of the population, perhaps, as upon climate, if we judge by these methods. We have already shown that the population of the Southern and Western States, is a *young population*, and, therefore, it is impossible that a large proportion of the deaths, should be in very advanced life. A larger proportion, in tables of this kind, above seventy years, as seen in New-Hampshire, Connecticut and European countries, does not prove those climates to be most favorable to human life. In Boston, for example, the proportion of deaths in early life, have increased for the last thirty-five years, and the proportion of advanced ages have diminished. The Charleston tables given, are more favorable for longevity, than those of Boston at any period, though many considerations should be examined, before positive conclusions are drawn.

THIRD METHOD.—*By ascertaining the proportion per cent, of persons surviving specified ages, but who die before the next specified age.*—This mode of ascertaining the law of mortality from the deaths alone, is more accurate than either of those before mentioned in the opinion of Mr. Shattuck; and taking the only data which we have from Charleston, viz: the last six years, this method is as favorable as the others, for the longevity of Charleston. It is found by dividing the number that died between two specified ages, by the number that survived the first mentioned age. The table below will show the number in Charleston, that survived each period, and the number and proportion, per cent, that died before the next period. For example, 2427, survived the age of 5 years, and of these 150 died before they reached the age of 10. Multiplying the 150 by 100, and dividing by 2427, will give 6,13 per cent, or the ratio which one bears to the other—the same method of calculation will show the proportion that died in each of the periods of life. This table for Charleston, includes Whites and Blacks; and as the deaths of the whites during these six years, were one in 58,12, while the blacks were 1 in 44, we may conclude that the estimates in this table are too high for the white population.

AGE.		Number surviving and dying in Charleston.	In each 100 surviving, there died before the next specified age.	BOSTON.
Under	1,	3569		
Dying under	1,	659	18,43	20,80
Surviving	1,	2910		
Dying before	5,	483	16,59	
Surviving	5,	2427		
Dying before	10,	150	6,13	3,58
Surviving	10,	2277		
Dying before	20,	239	10,49	10,80
Surviving	20,	2038		
Dying before	30,	420	20,60	26,83
Surviving	30,	1618		
Dying before	40,	395	24,41	31,71
Surviving	40,	1223		
Dying before	50,	372	30,41	31,95
Surviving	50,	851		

Longevity in reference to Life Insurance. 143

Age	Number Surviving and dying in Charleston.	In each 100 surviving, there died before the next specified age.	Boston.
Dying before 60	262	30,78	32,85
Surviving 60,	589		
Dying before 70,	231	39,21	42,00
Surviving 70,	358		
Dying before 80,	185	51,67	63,95
Surviving 80,	173		
Dying before 90,	112	64,74	86,17
Surviving 90,	61		

FOURTH METHOD.—*By ascertaining the average age at death.*—This has often been taken as a standard for comparing the health and longevity of different places, and though affording very valuable information, in an old settled country, which is little disturbed by emigration and immigration, it is not at all applicable to countries differently situated. Wherever there is a predominance of early life in a population, the average duration of life, (judging from bills of mortality,) will be low, and *vice versa.* The average duration of life, is found by adding together the particular ages of all that die, and dividing the aggregate by the whole number of deaths.

The population of Charleston was very stationary from 1830, to 1840, the whites having gained but 102, while the blacks lost 1130, and the average duration of life may perhaps on this account be more satisfactorily calculated than in any other town in the United States. According to the plan of calculating laid down by Mr. Shattuck, the average duration of life in Charleston, for the last six years, including all classes, was 30 years. I give below the average duration in different populations—with the fluctuations in several at different epochs:

Charleston,	30,09		
Boston,	from 21,43 to 27,85	England,	23,46
New-York,	" 19,69 to 26,15	London,	27,00
Philadelphia,	" 22,01 to 26,25	Liverpool,	20,00

FIFTH METHOD.—*By ascertaining the proportion which the number that died, bears to the number of the living at each specified age.*—This is no doubt the most correct standard of comparison between different places. If we know for example, how many there are living in the population of different places of any specified age, say between 5 and 10 years, or between 70 and 80, and we ascertain how many die at each specified age, we can easily calculate the proportion of the dead to the living, and compare the per centage. Such calculations would be very satisfactory, but there are no data by which a comparison of any two cities in the United States can be made. In Charleston, the census has been taken at intervals of 10 years, and the United States Census, (the only one taken,) classifies the whites and blacks differently; and lastly, the Register in his report, throws the ages and colors into one confused mass. There can be little doubt, from the results of the four preceding *methods*, that the fifth would be equally favorable to Charleston; but I shall not fatigue the reader with any calculations on this plan, which from the insufficiency of data, could only be approximative, and therefore indecisive.

Though the ratio which the gross annual mortality bears to the whole population, is not alone conclusive evidence of the health of a place, yet the fact is both interesting in itself, and important in connexion with others. I will give below the mortality of several town and countries.

DEATHS.		WHITES.	BLACKS.
Boston, 1811 to 1815, one in 47,5	Charleston, 1830, one in 39,45	40,00
Philadelphia, 1821 to 1830, one in 38,	" 1831, " 46,69	37,93
" " " whites, 42,	" 1832, " 51,91	55,35
" " " colored, 21,	" 1833, " 55,00	55,75
England 1839 to 1842, one in 45,	" 1834, " 42,14	44.16
France, 1810 to 1842 " 42,	" 1835, " 43,12	46,44
Austria, 1839 to 1841 " 33,	" 1836, " 40,68	19,64
Prussia, 1839 to 1841 " 38,	" 1837, " 47,37	46,79
Russia, 1842, " 38,	" 1838, " 18,30	33,00
London, " 37,38	" 1839, " 29.93	39.00
Birmingham, " 36,79	" 1840, " 50.76	46.64
Sheffield, " 32,92	" 1841, " 65.15	44.80
Leeds, " 37,73	" 1842, " 50.30	47.85
Bristol, " 32,38	" 1843, " 60.88	32.98
Manchester, " 29,64	" 1844, " 69.30	43.36
Liverpool, " 28,75	" 1845, " 52.96	48.54

This table for Charleston, commences at the period of the census of 1830 (since which time, the population has varied little,) and embraces sixteen years, which I have divided into three periods; the mortality is given for each period.*

* The following facts are taken from Volume 1st 1842, "Pritchard's Physical History of Mankind," and are very significant as to the question of acclimation, in climates far worse than those of our southern cities.

In Batavia in 1805, Europeans died	1 in, 11
" " " " Slaves "	1 in, 13
" " " " Chinese "	1 in, 29
" " " " Javanese, viz; *natives*	1 in, 40
In Bombay, 1815, Europeans died	1 in, 18
" " " Mussulmen	1 in, 17
" " " Parsees (natives,)	1 in, 40

Here we see the *natives* of these extreme climates, subjected to no greater mortality, than those of most parts of Europe. In Havana, the M. Moreau de Jonnés informs us, the mortality is one in 33 including all classes, and we know there must be a large per centage of foreigners.

It would seem that the ratio of mortality amongst the *whites* from 1830 to 1840, in Philadelphia was less than the preceding ten years, being, according to his calculations one in forty-six.

	WHITES.	BLACKS.	
1830 to 1834, one in	47,03	46,63	
1835 to 1839, " "	35,88	36,97	cholera and yellow fever period.
1840 to 1845, " "	58,21	44,03	

This table is favorable to the salubrity of Charleston, when we remember that in the second period (1835 to 1839) there were two epidemics of yellow fever, and one of Asiatic cholera; the former of which, attacked the unacclimated whites, and the latter, chiefly the blacks. Excluding the deaths from these causes, which is fair in estimating the effect of the climate on the acclimated whites and on the blacks, the mortality would be as low as in the other periods. The mortality for the last six years is perhaps not an unfair test, as the population was stationary and acclimated in a much greater proportion than in former years. From 1820 to 1830, the population increased about six thousand, and there were, of course, a great many foreigners thrown into the place during that time.

Charleston, like all our towns, both northern and southern, as it becomes more extended, better paved, better drained, more cleanly, (and the surrounding country also more dry,) becomes more healthy. There can be little doubt, that with her present police, if all immigration were cut off, she would continue almost exempt from yellow fever, and to a great extent from other fevers.

When we take into consideration the facts, that yellow fever attacks the unacclimated only—that it is only the better classes who apply for Life Insurance or annuities—that their tables of mortality include all classes, and that in all countries the lowest mortality is seen in the better classes, it seems clear that the tables of mortality for the last six years in Charleston, may be assumed as a safe basis for estimating the probabilities of life in Charleston, Mobile and New-Orleans.

The facts I have given, I hope, will receive the serious consideration of Northern Life Insurance Companies; my belief is, that no good reason exists for charging one per cent more on southern risks, where the applicants live in the seaport towns, and are acclimated, and if these companies will select faithful agents, and competent, honest, medical examiners, the result will prove the correctness of these opinions.

The medical examiners are now paid too little to make the office an object, and I would suggest that their compensation should be made, an insurance on their lives for some fixed amount, which would be forfeited if their risks were badly selected.

The statistics I have given, are not as complete as could be desired, but I hope this article may be received as a contribution towards the ends in view, and serve to stimulate others to further inquiry.

REPORT TO THE LOUISIANA STATE MEDICAL SOCIETY ON THE METEOROLOGY, VITAL STATISTICS AND HYGIENE OF THE STATE OF LOUISIANA

E[dward] H. Barton

REPORT

TO THE

LOUISIANA STATE MEDICAL SOCIETY,

ON THE

METEOROLOGY,

VITAL STATISTICS AND HYGIENE

OF THE

State of Louisiana.

BY E. H. BARTON, A.M., M.D.,

President of the Medical Society of the State of Louisiana; Permanent Member of the National Medical Association of the United States
Former Professor of the Theory and Practice of Medicine and Clinical Practice in the Medical College of the University
of Louisiana; Doctor of Medicine and Surgery of the Royal University of Havana, etc. etc. etc.

TO WHICH IS ADDED

AN APPENDIX,

Showing the Experience of Life Insurance Companies in Louisiana,
With Tables of Mortality for the use of such Companies,

And the Laws of Probability of Life (English Calculation);

ALSO, THE EXPERIENCE OF THE LONDON LIFE INSURANCE OFFICES, ETC.

BY H. G. HEARTT,

Actuary of the Mutual Benefit Life and Fire Insurance Company of Louisiana, and
Actuary of the British Commercial Life Insurance Company, of London.

New Orleans:

PRINTED AND PUBLISHED BY DAVIES, SON & CO.,

57 CAMP STREET.

1851.

Entered according to act of Congress, in the year 1851, by
HENRY GILBERT HEARTT,
In the Clerk's Office of the District Court of the Eastern District of Louisiana.

NEW ORLEANS, *March 27th, 1851.*

E. H. BARTON, A. M., M. D.:

Dear Sir:—The immense importance of correct Statistics of the Mortality of the City of New Orleans and the State of Louisiana, that comparison may be made with that of other Cities and States, in order to remove the unfavorable impression existing in regard to the health of this section of the Union, has induced us to request a publication of your very able and elaborate lecture on that subject, delivered before the Medical Society of the State of Louisiana, and upon the data of which you have bestowed so many years of observation and labor, making it an important and invaluable work of reference. Had more attention and publicity been given heretofore to Statistics, the growth of our City and State would have been more rapid, its population larger, and the sense of security of health would have caused also the retention of capital within its borders.

The want of correct statistics of mortality has been severely felt both here and in Europe, and its importance is further manifest, as it is only from such information that those institutions, created to alleviate the wants of families deprived of their natural supporters—Life Insurance Companies—can make the requisite mathematical calculations whereby the just rates of premium of life insurance and annuities can be established with reference to the Southern States; and in order that facilities may be given for the furtherance of this object, we renew our hope that you will favor us with a copy of your Report for publication, and remain, with high respect,

A. D. CROSSMAN,	S. J. PETERS,	ISAAC T. PRESTON,
J. H. CALDWELL,	JAMES ROBB,	ISAAC JOHNSON,
J. BALDWIN,	PETER CONREY, JR.	WM. FRERET,
LEONARD MATTHEWS,	JOHN HAGAN,	PIERRE SOULE,
C. C. SNETHEN,	JOHN A. DOUGHERTY,	ALFRED HENNEN,
H. G. HEARTT,	H. C. CAMMACK,	THEODORE CLAPP,
THOS. A. ADAMS,	WM. M. GOODRICH,	E. JENNER COXE, M.D.,
THOS. SLOO,	R. M. DAVIS,	E. H. CARMICHAEL, M.D.
E. L. GOOLD,	B. STILLE, JR.	HOWARD SMITH, M.D.,
T. B. THORPE,	SAMUEL WOLFF,	R. BEIN, M.D.,
R. F. CANFIELD,	J. THAYER,	G. W. SMITH,
BENJAMIN FLORANCE,	JOHN CLAIBORNE,	EDW. W. SEWELL.

NEW ORLEANS, *April*, 1851.

GENTLEMEN:

I have been honored with your note, requesting a copy of the report I made to the Louisiana State Medical Society, on the subjects of the Meteorology, Vital Statistics and Hygiène of the State, for publication. Though by no means insensible to its many imperfections, yet I must hope it will not wholly fail of service in the cause of life and health, since it has met the approval of persons of your position and intelligence; and with your leave, therefore, I WILL DEDICATE IT TO THE MUNICIPAL AUTHORITIES OF THE CITIES OF NEW ORLEANS AND LAFAYETTE, for whose enlightened consideration and judgment, its facts, principles and suggestions, were mainly designed.

Grateful for your approbation, and very obliging expressions,

I remain, gentlemen,

Most respectfully,

Your obedient servant and fellow citizen,

E. H. BARTON.

CONTENTS.

	PAGE
I.—METEOROLOGY, the agent in secondary causes — enumerated	8
Influence of temperature on the flowering of plants — ditto on disease	9
Hydrographical division of the State; amount inundated and subject to inundation	10
Instincts explained through meteorological conditions	12
Epidemics always connected with remarkable meteorological conditions	12
Meteorological and epidemic cycles the same; ditto of notable vegetable productions and animal migrations	13
The hygrometric state of the atmosphere, influence on health, how it acts	14, 15
Protective power of Lake Pontchartrain, difference in the climate of opposite banks of the Mississippi	15
Effect of a calm or stagnant atmosphere on health—probable cause of goitre and cretinism	16
The remarkable fatality of gorges or deep hollows in this and neigboring States, accounted for	16
The effect of winds and evaporation in lowering the temperature of the body, and in what ratio	17
Influence of the weight or pressure of the atmosphere, as indicated by the Barometer, on the body:	
1st. The effect of a very light atmosphere, what diseases prevalent where this exists, as exemplified in Mexico, etc.	18
2d. Remarkable influence of a greatly increased weight, as exhibited in some mines in France	18
How far is it in our power to influence meteorological conditions	18
The true estimate of the temperature of a climate to be derived from the temperature of the dew-point	16-20
II.—VITAL STATISTICS, ETC.—Why unfortunate for our sanitary showing, the taking the census at this period:	
1st, The Eastern district, remarkable salubrity of—2d, Western district, why less so	21
On what depends the permanent prosperity of the city; importance of knowing our actual condition	22-24
Reputation of New Orleans abroad; consequences of so long concealing or being ignorant of our situation	Ib.
Difference of mortality of city and country, cause of	25
Difficulty of detecting impure air, but by its effects — illustrations	26
Why the actual mortality of the city from the population *de facto*, is to be considered the true sanitary state	27
Can there be any real permanent acclimation, where the condition on which it depends is not stationary	28

CONTENTS.

	PAGE
When commenced the obscurity or doubt of the acclimating power of yellow fever	29
Is it possible for an acclimating disease to occur in a native, as a prerequisite for immunity against itself! the absurdity of such a proposition.	30
Proofs that the true malignant yellow fever is departing from among us—is blending itself with the ordinary diseases of the country	30
Individual habits of greater protective power than any acclimation	31
The effect of sanitary regulations in preventing yellow fever, amply demonstrated	32
Their effect in keeping the plague out of Egypt for centuries, contrasted with its return of late years, and the palpable causes pointed out; great mortality among the natives.	33
The evident connection of city mortality with physical changes, as exhibited during the last sixty years	34

III.—To what causes are to be attributed the insalubrity of this city; the actual calculated amount of organic matter putrifying and contaminating the air we breathe; bad air, and what produces it 35
Bad water; how injured; the great capacity of water to absorb deleterious gases, and whence derived 36
The importance of the proofs derived from science in explaining sanitary regulations 36
The effect of habits in a warm climate; temperance; influence of bad milk.. 37
Are the ills under which we suffer remediable? the great remedy, SEWERS; their absolute necessity; facility of making them; what they accomplish.. 38
The inapplicability of our present system of privies in our low soil, and why; how remedied 39
The necessity of covering our draining canals, and exclusion of light, different effects of stagnant and running waters 39
What kind of pavement required in this soil; duties of health wardens 40
The planting of trees in our squares and streets; how they act in purifying the air 40
Explanation of the principles of health and disease on the known laws of vital action 41
The direct effect of a high rate of mortality on the prosperity of the city 42
Important deductions from the foregoing data 42
Whence have arisen the popular errors in relation to the salubrity of the city. 43
That excuse, ignorance, exists no longer; all difficulties surmountable; the indispensable importance of putting the sanitary condition on a par with other cities, so as to compete with them for the trade of the country 44
Value of a knowledge of the connection of meteorological science with every day facts — with health — with agriculture 45
Importance of a registry law—of statistical records; how much we have been retarded by our past ignorance of them; illustration of what occurred at Liverpool 46
To what extent it has been demonstrated that the salubrity of a place can be improved by sanitary measures, and how far they are required here; proof that New Orleans not always sickly; that it has not arisen necessarily from climate or position, but from our neglect of sanitary measures entirely under our control 47
The true incubus that has been paralysing the slumbering energies of this community 47

CONTENTS.

PAGE

The actual average annual amount of moisture, number of grs. in a cubic foot, drying power, etc., three times a-day, shown for a long series of years; see table A............................ 48

The amount of moisture, drying power of each wind blowing over New Orleans; see table B.................................. 49

The prevalent wind of each month and season at New Orleans, on a long average of years; see table C. 49

The mortality of the city of New Orleans since 1787, with the ratios, the relative proportion dying at the Charity Hospital, and the dates of great physical changes in and about the city—table D............................... 50

Statement of the number of free and slave population, as well as the number of deaths from Cholera and other diseases, in the parishes of the Western District of Louisiana, as taken by the assistant marshals, and returned to the United States Marshal, under the census act of 23d May, 1850—table E... 51

Statement of the number of dwelling houses, free and slave population, as well as the number of deaths from Cholera and other diseases, in the respective parishes of the Eastern District of Louisiana, as taken by the different assistant marshals, and returned to the United States Marshal, under the census act of 23d May, 1850—table F. 52, 53

EXPLANATION.—The true interpretation of acclimation (intended as a note to page 31); its philosophy illustrated; so far as proved, is a meteorological condition 54

APPENDIX.—Result of the experience of life insurance companies in New Orleans; difference in mortality between blacks or whites reversed by them; illustrating the facility of preserving life here by care; great profits from life insurance resulting 56

Mutual Benefit Life and Fire Insurance Company of Louisiana.—A tabular view of the results of life insurance, as exemplified by the experience of this office, from its commencement to 1st April, 1851, a period of one year and nine months... 58

Mutual Benefit Life Insurance Company, Newark, New Jersey.—A tabular view of the results of life insurance, as exemplified by the experience of the Agency at New Orleans, from November, 1848, to June 1, 1851, a period of three years 59

Table of the rate of mortality at Carlisle, England............................ 60

Table showing the probabilities of the duration of human life at all ages from 10 to 97, deduced from the experience of the Equitable Insurance Company, of London 61

New rate of mortality in England.—A table, exhibiting the law of mortality amongst assured lives, according to the combined town and country experience of life offices, deduced from 62,537 assurances, under the superintendence of a committee of eminent actuaries, in London..................... 62

Table, showing the disorders (as certified to the court of directors) of which persons assured by the Equitable Society have died during thirty-two years, from the 1st of January, 1801, to the 31st of December, 1832 63

Table of comparative expectations of life in England.—Showing the expectation or average duration of life, deduced from eight original tables, prepared under the superintendence of a committee of eminent actuaries, and compared with the Carlisle, Equitable and Northampton tables............ 64, 65

CONTENTS.

Seventh Census.—Table showing the population of the United States, with the apportionment of Representatives 66

CHART No. I, illustrating the climate of several parts of the State, of the rainy seasons in four sections of the State, of the different temperatures of New Orleans in 1808 and '50, accounted for; the average monthly dew-point line here for a series of years, and below the average mortuary line from 1817 to 1850, showing healthiest and sickliest months 67

CHARTS Nos. II. and III. exhibit the different influences of the climate on color and on sex of same age 68, 69

ERRATA.

Page 7—Last line but one, for 'and' read *as*.

" 9—For 'and,' first word on the page, read *we shall*.

" 54—In fifth line from top, for 'fiscal' read *final*.

" 56—Second line from top, for 'Mutual Benefit Insurance Company,' read *Mutual Benefit Life and Fire Insurance Company*.

" 56—Seventeenth line from top, after 'and,' add *I*.

REPORT

ON THE

METEOROLOGY, VITAL STATISTICS AND HYGIÈNE

OF THE

STATE OF LOUISIANA.

Read before the Medical Society of the State of Louisiana, 7th March, 1851.

GENTLEMEN:

On our first organization, I had the honor to be appointed chairman of the Committee to report on the important subjects of the Meteorology, Vital Statistics and Hygiène of this State. On accepting that conspicuous post, I was not unaware of the sterileness of the field I had to work in — of the vast amount of toil to be bestowed to garner up fruits worthy of the Society, such as would fulfil the expectations, nay the *requirements* of science at this enlightened period of the world. I knew from many years' experience, that neither meteorology nor vital statistics were sufficiently prized by most of our cotemporaries here; that, consequently, but few records were kept of them. I shall now lay before you the result of my labors, imperfect though they be, and as our predecessors have signally failed in the performance of their duty — the scantiness of the materials left behind them must disarm criticism I should think, and leave me fair claims to your indulgence.

I. I commence the report at the fountain head — Meteorology; for these two subjects of Vital Statistics and the condition of the atmosphere have the direct influence of cause and effect impressed upon them. I wish to call your attention primarily to this connection, and we shall be the better enabled then to understand the nature of each, and appreciate our true position. In the great range of secondary causes, through which the influence of Deity is felt, meteorology is doubtless one of the mighty agents by means of which it is experienced. The subject is *attractive*, as its investigation unfolds the great laws of our Creator; it is *important*, for we cannot understand the great principles of climate and of health while ignorant of it; and it is *interesting* to us, for not a tree unfolds its leaves, nor a blossom expands its petals, nor the great science of agriculture, upon which we depend for our daily sustenance, is cultivated, without unfolding the truths and the science of meteorology. Whether, then, we are freezing under polar snows — scorching under tropical heats, or fanned by the zephyrs of milder regions, it so directly influences all, as to establish the popular belief (in which every man of science concurs), that it has a large share in most of our enjoyments, and materially influences nearly all our ailments. In a southern country, then, where a high range of temperature imparts to man an exalted sensibility, I may be pardoned for inviting your special attention to it.

The application of meteorological science — to the explanation of its influence on the vegetable and animal creation, and on man himself — the different races of man, — on the healthy and diseased condition, — is too extensive to be entered upon on the present occasion, or, indeed, upon any occasion within the proper compass of a single lecture. I can give but a very meagre sketch of the vast subject allotted to me. Vegetable and animal geography is one of the most captivating studies of the vast field of animated nature; but how much more important is that of man — influenced as he is in every latitude by these conditions; but to our profession belongs the speciality of its influence on his health — or *medical geography*. The why and wherefore that plague should exist in one country and yellow fever in another; — that Goitre should exist in Alpine regions, and Plica in Poland; — that Barbadoes leg should prevail in the Antilles and Beriberi in Ceylon; — that Matlazahuatl in Mexico and leprosy in Cuba, and that cholera should not pass the Equator, nor the yellow fever until last year, etc., etc., are as curious as they are well-established facts, showing the different influences of climate upon man. In the more highly advanced condition of this interesting science, and probably be enabled to explain the *modus operandi* of this influence, and thus be empowered to turn such knowledge to our benefit. Is not every thing to be expected from its progress, when we state to you that a French mathematician has demonstrated that a flower will bloom when the sum of the squares of the daily mean of temperatures reaches a certain point from the last freeze of winter! and that it has been ascertained that the common lilac blooms when this sum reaches 7607° of Fahrenheit's thermometer, and it has been already proved in relation to the recurrence of yellow fever of Philadelphia, in a series of years from 1793 to 1817, embracing many epidemics, that it occurred in no year when the average thermometer at 3 o'clock was under 79° during the summer, and that the extent and malignancy of the disease was proportioned to the extent in which it exceeded that height;—and that the average temperatures of June and July at that period governs the season in relation to health, insomuch that if, by the 1st of August in any year, the average shall be below that degree, we should feel full confidence that during that season yellow fever will not occur! In relation to this country, although this precise degree does not apply, (in an examination I have made of some nineteen years), yet the principle that the salubrity of the city greatly depends upon the elevation of temperature is fully borne out; and this does not at all detract from the value of the experience derived from what occurred at Philadelphia, for during the period under notice there was a more or less stationary and fixed condition of things in Philadelphia, while here almost everything has been in the transition state, and that though it is one of the most important agents influencing our sanitary condition, it is not the only one. These important statements evince the interest and value to be attached to the study of this department of science, and that it is a duty we owe to society, to the profession, and to our wants and enjoyments, to cultivate it.

I now present to the Society digested records of asmospherical conditions in this State for the last 30 years, made by myself, viz., of 12 years in West Feliciana; of 18 years in this city; of the journal kept by the scientific Lafon, for 1807, 1808 and '10 and 1819, here — of the parish of Rapides for the last 20 years, kept by a most worthy gentleman, Major P. G. Voorhies; and also the quantity of rain that has fallen during the last five years in the parish of Plaquemine, by Thomas Morgan, Esq. All these records have been carefully digested, out of which I have constructed Chart No. 1, illustrative, by comparison, of the climate of Louisiana in its different sections.

There are causes influencing our meteorological condition, which, in a proper estimate of our climate, we cannot overlook. I allude to the great modifying power of *large inland bodies of water* upon it. I am indebted to my friend, Professor Forshey, for the interesting computation. The whole area of the State of Louisiana is . . . . 48.972 square miles:
Of this—.
Marsh alluvion, west of delta (or
  Vermillion river) . . . . . 2.880   "
Mississippi delta, south of Red river
  (Lyell's limit of delta) . . . 12.514   "
Mississippi delta, north of Red river
  (within Forshey's delta) . . . 3.420   "
Red river alluvion above Avoyelles, 1.656   "
Ouachita   do. above Bœuf river, .900   "

    Making an aggregate, including
      flat lakes, of . . . . . . 21.370   "

All this is not constantly under water—but it is so more or less, and *constantly* subject to it. This does not include the alluvions of the smaller streams, and some, he admits, may have been reclaimed by levees. He farther states, that of the whole alluvion, there is uncultivable more than half, say 12,000 square miles, including shallow lakes.

You see, then, that about *one-eighth* of the State is constantly under water, and that more than *two-fifths* of it are subject to inundation. That this vastly influences its *thermal* as well as its *hygrometrical* condition in an annual average temperature of between 60° and 70°, and latitude between 29° and 33°, is too palpable to dwell upon,—indeed we know that it is so, and that if the hygrometrical is enhanced by it, its thermometrical is much lowered. Such I believe to be the fact in relation to contiguous territory, and that the climate of Louisiana is much milder and more equable from these causes, than large portions of Texas that are much to the south of us.

With these preliminary data, I propose now to enter upon a somewhat discursive examination of some of the most interesting arcana of nature unfolded by this beautiful science. Not only man, but all animal and vegetable creation is controlled by it. But little examination and reflection will be needed to convince us that it is through the laws of meteorology that the Deity acts (by secondary causes) in controling the actions and destiny of all animated nature.

That the qualities of the medium in which we live should produce disease, when there are great vicissitudes, when we are subjected to them under conditions we are not accustomed to, or when the system shall have acquired increased susceptibilities from other influences, is not at all extraordinary. In fact, it seems to be in precise accordance with the common sentiments of mankind. Medical men, (before the laws of meteorology were understood,) refining upon this universal assent, deeming it too vulgar, or not sufficiently recondite for the mysteries of scientific faith, thought proper to ascribe to another agency the production of the great mass of human maladies. Of the many wonderful powers of this supposititious agent, (miasm,) with attributes certainly incompatible with any known agent, I have nothing to do now; I only call your attention to some of the *sensible properties* of the atmosphere—to show that these qualities, so common as to be passed by almost unnoticed, are of the greatest importance in the preservation of our health, and that, together with personal indulgences and some hygiènic conditions, to be hereafter adverted to, most of the conditions productive of a pathological state are fulfilled. Confining ourselves, then, to the tolerably well demonstrated certainties of science, the cultivation of the profession and the advancement of our art, will be cotemporaneous with the alleviation of human suffering, and we shall be rewarded at each forward step in our career by witnessing the gratifying progress we have made.

Upon inferior animals which have not been endowed with this intelligence, or capacity, there has been vouchsafed a power that is an ample substitute for it, in those unerring instincts that urge them to provide for ordinary, as well as extraordinary, seasons—that teaches the beaver to prepare, by an additional story to his retreat, *months beforehand*, for a great overflow,—and the bee to lay up in *the autumn* for a *lengthened winter*. Surely this must be by and through some meteorological condition made known to them through their senses—as yet, so far beyond the reach of scientific certainty;—nay, man borrows information from the birds of the air and beasts of the field, foretelling approaching changes in the atmosphere, and his boasted science is nothing in these respects when compared with the power possessed by the inferior animals to guard their lives from danger. Without this conservative power, probably no race of animals could survive a single generation;—one would die of excessive heat, for which they were not duly prepared; another, from undue exposure to excessive cold; one by the hurricane they now scent at a distance; another prepares for the flood, that otherwise would destroy all exposed to it, and early providence prepares for a scarcity that must result from a condition that is to cause it; nay, we have seen the forest deserted by the feathered tribe, and the heavier beasts retreat to their most retired fastnesses on the approach of pestilence, and only return when it has subsided. That all this is communicated to them, as a strictly conservative power, through some meteorological influence, I do not doubt. That they influence man in the same way, is equally probable. Probably no general fact is more universally observed than the connection of great devastating epidemics with remarkable distemperatures of the air, unusual droughts, or deluges, great extremes of heat or cold, continued calms, or winds blowing for a long time from unusual quarters, hurricanes, etc.—nay, whatever has been unusual in the elemental conditions, so has varied the health of man—indeed, of inferior creation, too, for they have their epidemics as well as man. Astrology ascribed them to the condition and attraction of the heavenly bodies, and various have been the conjectures and superstitions of man in relation to it. The 'constitution of the atmosphere' for good or for ill, with whatever term it has been clothed, has exacted the general credence of mankind.

It is a curious fact in corroboration of this statement, that these meteorological zones or conditions occur in cycles of tolerable regularity, in periods of about seventeen years. So have been the occurrence of great epidemic visitations—the recent cholera and other disastrous diseases are well-known exemplifications of it. Such lustra, and of about the same duration, have been palpably recognised in agricultural pursuits—in the return of good or bad crops—of the cane dying and being reproduced every seventeen years; and in the animal creation, in the visitations of locusts, the flight of pigeons, etc. By-and-by the returns will be more exact, the coincidence more clearly shown, the law established, or it will be abandoned. The spirit of philosophic research is now abroad, and the lovers of truth will assuredly find it.

Since the birth of meteorology, (and it has been a very slow and tardy parturition,) as it unfolded its treasures, as successive data have been recorded, comparisons been instituted, diseases have been ascribed to one or the other of the changes that have been noted. Certain maladies are known to predominate during certain seasons, and these are characterised by variations of heat and cold; and so of the different climates, north and south. The most remarkable characteristic, and what has earliest struck the attention of mankind, has been the duration of certain temperatures. It was, however, soon seen that variations of temperature alone were not sufficient to account for all the different diseases prevailing in certain seasons and climates, for when these were the same, the influence on the health of man was very different. More or less rain was found to have its influence; so was the condition of the winds; and so of atmospheric pressure. These still not satisfying inquiry into the causes of the influences we experienced, the *hygrometric* condition was investigated, and it was soon seen that the greatest value was to be attached to it—that it was the only varying constituent of the atmosphere,* often independent of rain and temperature;† that it

---

* For it should be looked upon in that light, though not *technically* so.

† Extraordinary as this may appear to the scientific reader, my journal clearly demonstrates it, and confirms a theory on the subject now in the press, by Professor Espy.

readily accounted for most of the influences ascribed to miasm. In proportion, then, to the observation of atmospheric phenomena, so have been their connection with morbid condition. It is much to be regretted that scientific meteorology has advanced very slowly, and has not been made a part of medical education, as it should have been, cotemporaneous with pathology.

If man was perfect in his condition, and all hygiênic rules fulfilled, and we had the means of knowing *all* meteorological conditions, we should probably be enabled to explain through them his entire liability to disease, and then probably prevent or correct the greater part. Here, with a medium temperature throughout the year of about $67° \frac{43}{48}$, the winter mean being 54.48, the spring 73.56, the summer 79.38, and the autumn, 67.94, the range during the year rarely exceeding $50°$, it is clear that neither the average temperature, nor the extremes, should alone be highly detrimental to health. Doubtless this condition is much influenced by the alternations of land and water; it is thus less hot than if altogether dry, and less cold from the same cause. This condition thus favoring us with regard to temperature, is productive of another result, not so favorable in relation to the hygrometric condition. In Table A you will find the actual amount of moisture in the atmosphere, both on the thermometric and hygrometric scales, its elasticity, the number of grains of moisture in each cubic foot, and also the drying power, or force of evaporation, three times a-day, for each month in the year, for an average of a long series of years, furnishing a very correct estimate of the climate in these highly important particulars.

The *hygrometric* condition is less known and appreciated than any other, and probably more nearly influences our sanitary state and enjoyments. Its frequent and great changes are often mistaken for *thermometric* alterations; many persons, feeling the change they experience, are astonished, on looking, to find the stationary condition of this latter; and these changes are sometimes very great. So far as philosophical experiments have gone, hardly a doubt exists of the fact that the winds that have obtained their appellations (such as the simoon, kamsin, etc.) from the pestilences they have borne upon their wings, have derived their qualities mainly from their hygrometrical states;—one is loaded with vapor, saturates the atmosphere, prevents the decarbonizing power of oxygen on the blood, relaxes the system, increases the freedom of the secretions by which the blood is impoverished and kept prepared for the important purposes of life; while another, on the contrary, desiccates the blood, dries up the secretions by which it is depurated, and arrests vital action by rapidly depriving the system of the fluids requisite to sustain the organs in the due performance of their functions. In either excess, then, life is jeoparded, and much more than by mere extremes of temperature. This is clearly proved by the fact of the sickliest countries and seasons having the highest dew-point; that in elevated, or other regions, or at sea, where the highest salubrity is enjoyed, a medium hygrometric state is usually present, except when influenced by a prevalence of particular winds, that convey certain amounts of moisture with them. I think the present state of meteorological investigations will authorise me to announce these as *established facts.*

Table B furnishes you the *hygrometry* of the different winds blowing over New Orleans during an average of near eight years. They are doubtless much influenced by the remarkable manner in which the great delta is variegated with alternate expansions of land and water, viz., that all the northern winds, and even the western, have their dryness much decreased by blowing over large bodies of water; and my impression is, that Lake Pontchartrain will actually one day materially aid in protecting New Orleans from the violence of pestilences, by furnishing a moderate moisture to the atmosphere, and lessen that desiccating power that usually prevails at those periods when the swamps to the east and north-east of us are dried up. The modifying influence of a body of water of less than a mile in breadth, is conclusively shown by the difference between the two banks of the Mississippi river, where it runs east and west, the south side having a milder climate—vegetation earlier advances in the spring—the cane has a longer period to mature in autumn, and fruits that are occasionally cut off by the severity of weather on the north bank, are uninfluenced on the other.

I present you Table C, showing you what is the prevalent wind during each successive month and season, on an average of ten years.

On an inspection of Table B, you will observe how much the moisture is increased during a CALM—that here it always exhibits the maximum of moisture. This condition of atmosphere is, fortunately for us, very rare in this country, unless artificially produced. Stagnation in air or water, nay, in any form of vegetable or animal life, seems to be against the laws and will of Providence. In air, where it exists for any length of time, there is hardly comfort, health, or even life. There are but two places on the globe mentioned by travellers—'valleys of the shadow of death'—that cannot be visited by animated beings and returned from alive; places whitened by the bones of the victims of temerity, where, it is even said, that birds cannot fly over with impunity. In these positions, with a stagnant air, (and consequently high dew-point,) no change takes place, and it is in a position approximative to this that goitre and cretinism occur. There are deep ravines or gorges in the upper part of this and the adjoining States, near to which it is utterly unfit for man to reside, and especially at their outlets, (I speak from personal experience.) Occasionally, a body of air passes out of these hollows which is particularly injurious to the health of man. There, then, of course, with a stagnant air, is a high dew-point. Such, too, is the influence on health—and remarkably so in a warm climate, of living in houses that cannot be well ventilated, and having yards in which all the filth is located, where neither the light of heaven nor a breath of air can reach.

Stagnation in air or water is always more or less accompanied with impurity. Such, too, is the necessity of circulation in the great body of water which surrounds the globe, that an all-wise Providence has everywhere distributed it in currents, making it useful to its inhabitants, as well as man. Change, then, is the great law of being—it is essential both for purity and health.

The constant perflation which our position guarantees us, not only dries the country more rapidly, but cools the body down to the dew-point, or near it; certainly a most important, though unregarded, fact. From experiments instituted, it has been clearly proved that the quantity of fluid removed from the system is nearly three times as much in a moderate breeze, and upwards of four times as much in a fresh wind, as in a calm or stagnant state of the atmosphere.

But there is another condition of the atmosphere almost as much overlooked as the hygrometric, and probably as much so, in a hygienic point of view; I allude to the weight, or pressure of it, as indicated by the *barometer*. From the weight of the air being measured by mercury, which is so much heavier than air, (11,026 times,) the changes indicated by it are comparatively small. When the barometer is made of water, (which is only 815 times heavier than air,) the almost constant undulations and vibratory movements of the atmosphere are very apparent, and we can readily understand why more or less of this pressure or weight should influence us, not only in health, but disease. This will be better appreciated when we reflect that every square inch of our surfaces is exposed to a pressure of 14.6 ℔s. Allowing, then, the surface of a man's body, of the medium size, to be 15 square feet, or 2,160 square inches, he suffers the enormous pressure of 31536 ℔s., or more than fifteen tons! It is, nevertheless, passed by unnoticed by us ordinarily, because the pressure within and without are equal. Not so, however, with the *variations*, and, if we analyse them, they will appear immense. For instance, a fall or rise of $\frac{1}{10}$ of an inch (of the mercury) indicates a difference or removal of 100 ℔s. to the square inch; of $\frac{2}{10}$, of 200 ℔s.—not at all unusual in this country, though much more common to the north; a fall of $\frac{5}{10}$, of 500 ℔s.; of 1 inch, of 1000 ℔s.; of 3 inches, of 3000 ℔s., etc. When the barometer falls, instead of feeling 'light,' as we should by the removal of any other weight from us, our breathing becomes difficult, feeble, frequent, and often terminates in an asthmatic paroxysm; the pulse is quick and most compressible; hemorrhages often occur, with a tendency to fainting; the secretions scanty and easily suppressed, and, at length, with a farther and greater exposure, apathy supervenes; we feel sluggish, heavy and spiritless, owing to the excessive expansion of the fluids in the vessels; we experience the want of that tonicity which braces us up, and we denominate it, by a singular perversion of sense and language, 'a heavy atmosphere'! That such a condition of atmosphere should affect our healths is, on the least reflection, not at all extraordinary—and such is the fact. Illustrations in abundance could be furnished you—my time warns me to be content with one, and that relates to the City of Mexico. This large and magnificent capitol of that once wonderful people, is situated at an elevation of about 7.700 feet above the level of the sea, or our level, and, accordingly, disease is here modified by a pressure and elasticity due to a removal of near 15,000 ℔. weight, arising from a barometric pressure of little over 25 inches, or near half the atmospheric pressure. And what we should theoretically anticipate from this condition of things, is actually found to take place, and that the diseases of the *thoracic cavity*, with a few of the liver, (and these mostly of abscess,) and a large proportion of dropsies, contribute nearly 34 per cent. of the entire mortality, calculated from an aggregate of a series of years, most carefully, by myself.

Farther to illustrate my position of the more or less influence of the pressure of the atmosphere on our systems, I will mention another, but opposite, example, the results of some experiments made by M. Junot, and described by him in the *Archives Générales de Médicine*, to show the bracing and cheering influence of *condensed air* on the system. It was found that a person so exposed, breathes with increased facility; he feels as if the capacity of the lungs was enlarged—his respirations become deeper and less frequent—he experiences in the course of a short time an agreeable glow in his chest, as if the pulmonary cells were becoming dilated with an elastic spirit, while the whole frame receives at each inspiration fresh vital impulsion; the functions of the brain are excited, the imagination becomes vivid, the ideas flow with delightful facility, digestion is rendered more active, as after gentle exercise in the air, because the secretory organs participate immediately in the increased energy of the arterial system. These experiments were made on persons in a mine in France, where men worked with a pressure of three atmospheres. Upon many of them the first sensations were painful, especially upon the eyes and ears, but ere long they became quite reconciled to the bracing element. Old asthmatics here become effective operatives, deaf persons recover their hearing, while others are sensible to the slightest whisper. The latter phenomena doubtless proceeds from the strong pulses of the dense air upon the membrane of the drum of the ear. Men who descend to considerable depth in diving bells, experience a considerable augmentation of muscular energy; it infuses into the muscles such power, that they can easily execute double the work, without fatigue, which they are enabled to execute in the open air; they thereby acquire the power of bending over their knees strong bars of iron, which they would find quite inflexible by their utmost efforts, when drawn up to the surface.

From these statements of the effects of meteorological conditions — and they might be greatly enlarged — it is apparent to every one that their influence is very great. I now again invite your attention to Chart No. 1, giving a bird's-eye view of these variations, on *averages* of every month in the year (of course the *extremes* would exhibit them more palpably). There are two lines wherein are traced the temperatures for this city for every month in the year; and the Charts Nos. 2 and 3 will exhibit the mortality during the same period. No. 2 will show the different effects of the climate on RACES of the *same age*, (white and black) and No. 3, the direct effect on the mass monthly. Here, then, several facts are most clearly and palpably exhibited: first, the different mortalities for the different months; second, the modifying influence on the black and white race of the same age; third, the diverse effect on the different sexes of our own race, the cause of which I shall advert to hereafter. The slightest contemplation of these Charts will satisfy every one of the intimate bearing of meteorology (or climate) upon mortality.

Now, the important practical question arises, how far is it in the power of man so far to modify these conditions, when in excess, as to ameliorate their injurious influences. It is gratifying to state that much may be done in obeying the great command 'of subduing the soil and adapting it to the purposes of man;' by removing the forest growth, draining the swamps, and cultivating the soil, we lessen the amount of moisture, (which with us is of the greatest injury,) not only from the extent of area exchanging its moist, to a dry, condition, but we increase the perflation thereby, and hence, by increasing evaporation, (the drying power,) and lowering the dew-point, we actually lower the temperature. This has been really accomplished here in relation to temperature, for, by comparing Lafon's tables of average temperature for New Orleans in 1807, '10, with the temperature observed by me here, 1833–'50, the average is less by nearly 3°, while the extremes are less. Chart 1 contains these two lines of temperatures, for comparison. The same Chart embraces, also, the average monthly temperatures of West Feliciana and Rapides, and are so designated; while below is demonstrated the DRY and RAINY SEASONS of four different sections of our state. Three of these correspond, viz., those of New Orleans, Placquemine and Rapides; while that of West Feliciana, although an average of about 13 years, seems to have had *three* rainy seasons; it was then at a somewhat earlier period than of the three first, and may be considered in its *transition state*, being cleared of its forest growth mainly since that period; it has probably obeyed what is more likely to be a law of the climate in relation to other portions.

II. Let us proceed to the second branch of our subject— "The Vital Statistics and Hygiène of the State." The period adopted for taking the mortality of the State, with its census, has been an unfortunate one for Louisiana, for during the whole period embraced under the order to the marshals and their deputies for this enumeration, viz., the year ending in June, 1850, has been precisely one of those periodical cycles alluded to in the former part of this report as about the septemdecennial period for the return of epidemic cholera. Such has been the fact, and large mortality has resulted in the whole zymotic class (to which cholera belongs); for although I have been enabled to separate the cholera from the other mortality in most of the parishes, yet the mortality has been much larger in the congenerous diseases of that class, than usual; and many parishes of the western district of the State, (see table E),* where we know that the mortality is not in ordinary years more

---

* I am indebted to the politeness of Colonel Labuzan, deputy marshal, for most of this important and interesting table, and to C. Gayarré, Esq., Secretary of State, for the separate column of cholera in table E.

than one to one-and-a-half per cent. has been made, by this return, to show four, five, six, eight per cent., and upwards! This is to be deeply regretted, and the only remedy to be found is in the enactment of a registration law by the State legislature, through which the actual sanitary condition can be made known annually. From this somewhat sombre picture, let us turn to the Eastern District (see table F), which exhibits a degree of salubrity probably not surpassed on the globe. It will be observed, (for the aid of memory and observation) I have classed the parishes in both districts, into RIVER, SWAMP and UPLAND, according to their geographical location, at the foot of the table, and it will be seen that the average of the SWAMP parishes of Louisiana, which have heretofore been characterised, by those unacquainted with our State, as the dread and perennial abodes of disease and death, the mortality, (deducting cholera), has been less than one-half of one per cent. per annum (0.44), with the whites, and with it but $\frac{63}{100}$ of 1 per cent! In the river parishes it was a fraction over 1 per cent. (1.03); and with the upland, 1½ per cent. (1.57)! We should be amply satisfied with this showing, and it is the only answer that is required to the blasting and enduring criticisms upon the salubrity of the rural districts of this country, which have so long abused both popular and scientific credulity abroad. I am duly sensible that the country is much more healthy now than when first subdued to the purposes of culture; it then partook, with all new countries, of the maladies incident to a change from a state of nature. Its sanitary condition since has been constantly advancing, under the ameliorating hand of cultivation, and probably no part of our common country is more favored with this choicest of blessings. In comparing the western with the eastern districts under the classification I have adopted, it will strike you how different they are as to salubrity — how much more healthy the eastern are; it is easily explained: all agricultural countries are most sickly when first opened to cultivation; — the eastern have passed through that lustrum — the western are now suffering under it.

With this cheering view of the salubrity of our rural districts, let us come nearer home, to one where the improving hand of man, although it has done something (but for the most part incidentally), yet much remains to be done, that experience, reason and science most unequivocally point out as *indispensable* to our progressive advancement. Neither our geographical nor topographical position, nor climatural influences, discourage the hope nor the prospect, that with proper care we can approximate that degree of salubrity enjoyed by the country around us. The permanent prosperity of this city mainly depends upon the degree of salubrity that is to be attained and enjoyed by the *mass* of the inhabitants,—not the wealthy portion, merely, who can take the 'wings of the morning and fly to the uttermost parts of the earth,' but of those that are to live and toil here all the year long, and also of that large class who visit us not only for the purposes of business but of pleasure. The subject, then, is of the last importance to us, and upon its proper solution depends our future welfare and advancement. Railroads, canals, and steam lines, are certainly of great importance; I would not underrate them if I could, but their primary tendency is to make your mart but a GREAT FACTORAGE—a depot for the sale and interchange of commodities, which can be effected in a few months. If the mass cannot be reasonably sure of living here as long as elsewhere, these facilities will only increase that system of absenteeism which is now retarding, like a curse from God, the population and progress of a city blessed with natural advantages which no other city on either continent, possesses. Two great difficulties encompass this subject, the removal of which is absolutely essential to its thorough investigation: the first is the great error under which we have long labored in relation to our salubrity; and the second is, the procurement of the actual facts to ascertain what that condition has been. The first is palpably a preliminary, for it is obviously useless, if not hurtful, to attempt an improvement, when it is believed none is needed; and to apply a remedy where there is no disease, and especially if this shall be an expensive one. 'If ignorance is bliss, it were a folly to be wise.' Here, however, the reverse is the actual truth; and it requires some moral courage to disabuse a community of a long and deeply-cherished error. We hug our chains with delight, and stone the man who will attempt to convince us that they are but the chains of sciolism and ignorance, forgetful at the time that we but deceive ourselves, and that the world is not to be gulled at this enlightened epoch by our assertions, when unsupported by facts, and our self-complacency, when not based upon truth. Of the second, any one can convince himself who will undergo the arduous labor of seeking for such a record of births, deaths and marriages, as is kept by every other enlightened city of similar dimensions and importance. I trust, however, before the conclusion of this report, not only to prove to your satisfaction that you have long labored under a very serious error — one, in truth, very fatal to your prosperity, but that sufficient facts have been gathered, by years of research, to point out wherein it has existed, — enough to warrant the conclusion, that the 'conviction of an error' is, in this instance, at least equivalent 'to the establishment of a truth.'

The Vital Statistics of this city have been, until comparatively a recent period, almost untrodden ground: 'the horrid devastating epidemics' have been written of and described; the forbidden months, 'the dead season,' have hurried thousands from our midst upon the wings of wealth; catacombs of those who dared to tempt the lurid shores, or were destitute of the means of flight, have been long buried with their hopes, and been rapidly forgotten. The survivors alone have been counted; the dead have not been missed in the mighty throng that the love of thrift has brought to succeed them in the large spoils here offered to the industrious and enterprising, and the city has been characterised abroad as a great Golgotha, and signalised for its perennial pestilence. And what RECORD has been made of the *past*, for the benefit of the *future?* — *that future which to us is the present!* For more than fifty years this important entrepot has been in possession of a race believed to be the most intelligent and enterprising of all that dwell upon earth; yet they, in the great contest for mammon, have left but few records to tell us of that past, as a beacon and warning for the guidance of the future. The value of that knowledge will be appreciated, when we reflect that we grow wiser by degrees; that our present suffering depends upon our ignorance of the past; and to successive generations, the future can only be instructive, when the errors of the past are pointed out, and shunned as objects for our avoidance. To be sure, suffering is the chastisement, in the hands of Wisdom, out of which is often wrought the most eminent good. The effort, then, that will carry success with it, will show that the chastening and the love have gone together.

The statistical data forming the basis of this report have been the slow accumulation of years, nor can I answer for their entire reliability; but then they are the best established facts I could procure on the subject, and it becomes us, as professional men and philosophical observers, to scrutinise them closely,—if they are false, to prove them so; for it is not by *denying* them, that we can correct the insalubrious condition of this city. Let us obtain the *truth*, by all means. If insalubrious, let us, by patient investigation, and putting all the facts within our reach together, ascend to the *causes*, and correct them, if possible. This is the true mode of being a real friend to our country, and not by flattery and concealment of the truth; for in this way we only deceive ourselves. No one abroad gives credit to the oft-repeated assurances of the salubrity of the city; and its influence, so far as believed by us, is most fatal to our safety, for it only superinduces that self-satisfaction at our situation, and apathy and opposition to improvement, and particularly if expensive, that presents an effectual barrier to our advancement. Figures (that is, statistics) is a great leveller; they are inexorable; they have little respect for partialities or prejudices; they often deal harshly with theories and speculations; they serve to correct the extravagancies of the imagination, and are often the surest tests of truth. The theory that cannot abide numerical ratios from well-ascertained and properly recorded facts, advances us but little, nay, retards us, in our progress towards true and exact knowledge. By their means we are enabled to remove the proverbial taunts of which our profession is the 'scape-goat.' They must put an end, if anything can, to the false facts which have so long cast derision on the profession. This, if anything, must place our noble calling on the list of the exact sciences, and aid largely in the safety and duration of human life.

In a State like Louisiana, whose main population has been made up by immigration, and that mostly within the last thirty years, whose floating population has always been so large, and particularly in the cities and towns, (and there are no records to separate the native from the immigrant,) we are deficient in the main means, the basis, to acquire a knowledge of the effect of the climate upon health. This, however, is the less to be regretted, because the country is new—is constantly undergoing vast changes, which must, and always does, affect its sanitary condition.

You will have observed, in Table F, the ratios of mortality in the city and country are very different, and I could readily have furnished you extensive proofs of this general, and, indeed, universal fact. The causes are very obvious:—the population of the one lives in a crowded workshop, as it were, and breathes a confined and impure air; the population of the other spend the greater part of their time in, and breathe the pure air of heaven, where its impurities are diluted, scattered by the winds and oxydised in the sun, and where vegetation is constantly incorporating such elements as are noxious to man; while in cities, in proportion to density of population, there is constantly and insensibly thrown off an atmosphere of organic matter, which 'hangs over cities like a cloud,' slowly spreading, dispersed by the winds, and washed down by showers. 'It is a matter which *has lived*, is dead, has left the body, and is undergoing oxydation and decomposition into simpler than organic elements. The exhalations from sewers, church-yards, vaults, slaughter-houses, cess-pools, commingle in this atmosphere as polluted waters enter the Thames, (I am quoting from the report of the Registrar-General of England, but the same is equally, and, I will prove presently, more applicable to us,) and, notwithstanding the wonderful provision of nature for the speedy oxydation of organic matter in water and air, accumulate, and the density of the poison (for, in the transition of decay, it is a poison) is sufficient to impress its destructive action on the living, to receive and impart the processes of zymotic principles, to contaminate by a subtle, sickly, deadly medium, the people agglomerated in narrow streets and courts, down which no wind blows, and upon which the sun seldom shines.' It is to this that the high mortality of towns is owing,—living in and constantly breathing an atmosphere charged with decomposing matter, of vegetable and animal origin; and, however small the quantity, even beyond the reach of chemical tests, we have abundant proofs of their existence, besides their effects, from comparative conditions. 'Sulphuretted hydrogen and ammonia, and other gases, may be diffused in quantities so great as to be detected by the senses, or by chemical analysis, or so minute and inodorous as to escape detection, and, in either case, may be the cause of disease. Some idea may be formed of the almost infinite divisibility of matter diffused in the atmosphere, from the fact that the hound, in the chase, discerns the tract of man and animals by the odoriferous particles thrown off from their foot-prints, and that we detect the odor of musk, notwithstanding the single grain from which it proceeds was deposited twenty years previous, and has since been constantly diffusing its particles in the surrounding atmosphere. The experiments of Thenard and Dupuytren proved that birds perished when the vapors of sulphuretted hydrogen and ammonia exist in the atmosphere to the extent of a fifteen-thousandth part, and that dogs are deprived of life when the air they breathe contains a thousandth part, and that a man cannot live when the air he inspires is impregnated with a three-hundredth part, and suffers in a corresponding degree when a less proportion of these poisonous gases exist. Persons frequently fall dead when entering a well, vault, tomb, sewer, or other place filled with these gases, or with stagnated air, in which are diffused emanations from decomposing animal, vegetable or mineral substances.' Leibig, with all the appliances of the Giessen laboratory, cannot yet detect any difference between the pure air of the Alps and the air through which the hound can tell a horse, a fox or a man has passed, or the air which observation shows will produce small-pox, measles, scarlatina, whooping-cough, dysentery, cholera, influenza, typhus, plague.[*] Man himself cannot breathe the same air with impunity: every minute of every day he appropriates to the vitalization of his blood twenty-four cubic inches of oxygen, and supplies its place with twenty-four inches of carbonic acid gas. When present in large quantities, from whatever cause produced, carbonic

---
[*] General Report of the Board of Health of England.

acid gas is destructive of life. Charcoal burning in a close room is a familiar illustration.

Such, then, is the immediate cause of the difference between city and country; and we shall perceive presently whence they proceed, and how far they are removable. The great mass of mankind is ignorant that, with the tempting and fascinating allurements of a city life, they are constantly inhaling the poison and imbibing the draught which will shorten their days, because their attention is not drawn to them, and they leave it to others, whose duty it thus becomes to apply the proper remedies. The great difference that exists between the mortality of city and country is well known; it sometimes amounts to near forty per cent. The cause is quite as well established. The inhabitants of a city are constantly deteriorating in vitality, and in the course of years whole families frequently waste away and become exinct, from this and other causes, unless recruited by a union with others from the country; and it is well known, most large cities are so sustained and increase. I have no room for details.

Let us apply these principles to New Orleans; but we will first present you the facts as far as they could be procured, of our mortality here, as far back as 1787, with gaps which no industry of mine could fill up. Upon this we base our deductions, (see Table D). To make up this table, I have not been able to deduct from it the accidents, and the numerous causes of death other than *disease*, nor have I deducted the epidemics, or been able to ascertain what portion of the population, native or immigrant, have fallen victims; but I have taken the *whole mortality* as I procured it, and have computed the per centage as usual. If the showing is a bad one, the *greater will be the need to remedy it*, and it will be shown in the sequel that this is much in our power.

In a country whose population is mainly made up by immigration, and in which the great influence is mostly felt, the *actual mortality* that occurs in the population *de facto* is the one of real importance, and not its influence on the native; and it is of little practical importance now, to inquire what may be the effect of the climate on the native. There is little that is permanent in the condition of the country; it is, has been, and will be, for a long time, in what may be termed its TRANSITION STATE.

When most of the physical changes, as draining, clearing, canaling the country, with such paving, sewerage and policing, as is indispensable for a fair trial of the position, is made, it will be time enough to discuss the effect of a stationary condition, and by that time we shall, probably, be supplied with some records, better than opinions, as a foundation to speculate on. This is the more especially true, because, with the changes induced in the country by its reduction from a wild forest growth to a high cultivation, the health of man particularly suffers; for in either of the two extremes, of a state of nature and a general cultivation, there is general health, with exceptions easily explained. Hence, then, the actual mortality in the *statu quo* is sufficient for our purpose; in fact, we are limited to that, as there are no details of their separation, nor even if we had them would they be of much practical value, unless we had a distinct acclimating disease, putting the acclimated and the native on the same footing. But how is that possible in a physical condition, on which it depends, which is constantly changing? A mere reference to the dates of these great improvements, whose influence on health at the moment is generally considered injurious, however beneficial afterwards, will convince you that there has been no stationary condition, for any great length of time, in and about this city, for more than sixty years, but more particularly since the digging of the bank canals; from the excavation of the Canal Carondelet, in 1794,–'7, to the digging of the canals in our rear, to drain, and the draining and removal of the forest growth in our swamp, which was, in fact, only completed during the last year. The Table D has the dates of these improvements. Hence, then, the discussion of the existence or necessity of any specified acclimation is pretty much superseded; for it is very doubtful if there can be any acclimation in a city whose *status*, or condition, is not somewhat stationary,—whose essential climatural features (or at least those which so greatly influence health) are so constantly varying. It is my impression that there cannot, and such is the result of my experience and observation. Indeed, the whole subject of acclimation, or the effect of habituation to a country protecting the party from the endemic diseases of that country, has been much overrated. Such acclimation is not even pretended to be extended to northern climates, but why it should be limited to southern ones is not alleged. An examination into this subject, by the British army surgeons, both in the East and West Indies, shows that there exists no such protective influence. On the coast of Africa, no such immunity (nor in Egypt) is acquired,* and I am yet to be entirely satisfied that, of late years at least, such safety has been acquired here to any great extent, during the progress of the great physical alterations of which our city and neighborhood have been the theatre.

YELLOW FEVER, the great acclimating fever so called, (and it is doubtful whether there is any other, and none such has been alleged) was formerly easily characterized; its symptoms were less equivocal than they have been since, and no doubts were expressed in giving its appellation at an early period. For the truth of these statements, I must refer to the definite recollections of my cotemporaries of former times. The vast physical alterations to which I have reference, commenced to have more palpable progress but a few years previous to the division of the city, in 1835, and in 1836 there occurred a type of fever that the most experienced among us, at that time, were slow in christening as decided cases of yellow fever; and really there were numerous cases that we adjourned over the decision of until the subjects of them should be exposed to a fever of a more decided and unequivocal type. Ever since that period equivocal cases have been constantly occurring, and the more so of late years, so as to give rise to the question, often asked and discussed, of 'what is yellow fever?' and to the opinion expressed by several of our most experienced practitioners, that yellow fever often occurs in the same individual more than once, or, in other words, is no longer *a preventive of itself;* and hence, is no longer an acclimating

---

* I give the following table to show the difference in the mortality of different races during the plague at Alexandria in 1835:—

Negroes and Nubians	lost 84	per cent.	of their population.
Malays	" 61	do.	do.
Arabs (not soldiers)	" 55	do.	do.
Greeks	" 14	do.	do.
Jews, Armenians and Copts	" 12	do.	do.
Turks	" 11	do.	do.
Italians and others from the south of Europe	" 7	do.	do.
French, English, Prussians and Germans	" 5	do.	do.

disease; and that it occurs in the natives of the city, even at the earliest ages, (never alleged formerly); which, if true, settles that question. For the very idea that there is something specific required, arising from physical condition, to acclimate one to a place where an individual is *born, and has never left*, appears to me unnecessarily refined and entirely untenable. It has been expressed to me by some of our oldest inhabitants, those who have been observers of the disease twenty or thirty years ago, that it was no longer the same disease; that, in fact, the unequivocal malignancy and peculiar type which characterised it exists no longer; and this is most amply verified by the symptoms, aspect and history of the disease in its various stages, as seen and described by those who had witnessed it from 1804 to 1823, now in my library; and that for some years back it has been blending itself with the ordinary diseases of the country. I have elsewhere expressed this opinion, and have formed it after due deliberation.† Every now and then, we nevertheless meet with cases where there is no room for doubt, but they bear a very small proportion to the mass of cases which occur here every year.

This position is fully sustained by the record I now give, the result of an investigation into all the yellow fever years of which I could procure the details, and fortunately, after much research, I have been able to obtain those of the worst years. The disastrous year of 1847 may be considered an exception, and the remarkable mortality then may, in part, be attributed to the large temporary influx to our population, arising from a state of war, and 20,000 troops, with their proverbial recklessness, encamped for some time among us; and, also, that of later years, many

YEARS.	PER CENT. TO TOTAL MORTALITY OF THE YEAR.	RESULTS OF PERIODS.
1817	33.86	
1819	19.87	
1820	22.66	
1822	29.55	26.48
1829	35.71	28.13
1833	22.08	26.12
1839	22.45	
1841	29.84	
1842	10.78	19.74
1843	15.89	
1846	3.16	
1847	30.26	
1848	10.84	10.57
1849	7.79	
1850	1.33	

---
† Board of Health Report for 1849.

cases have been 'docketted' as yellow fever which would not have been so denominated in 1817,'22, etc. These valuable facts, taken in connection with what has been accomplished in other countries, (mentioned in a preceding part of this report,) and particularly in Egypt formerly, will fully bear me out in the opinion I have expressed, that, with the *completion of our physical improvements, yellow fever will have disappeared from among us.*

The facts—the painful, stubborn facts, which we can neither evade or deny, are, that for the last ten years our mortality has been upwards of 5½ per cent. per annum; and it is of a people who must be presumed to have had fair average constitutions, brought here, or raised here. They have died from *some cause* —they have died from *disease;* and it is immaterial whether it is called 'acclimating fever' under which they sunk, or intestinal, or pulmonary disease : it is the fact of death and loss to the public which is to be considered. Nor do I think it very material whether the mass of the mortality is of the recent arrivals, or not; it does not favor the argument, for, if they have been here but a very short period, the climate, or something, must be extremely lethiferous to have killed them so soon.

The term acclimation is very indefinite, so as to apply to records in civil life that can be of any use to the statistician. If it is confined to *yellow fever*, there is no record of it unless the subject falls a victim to it. There is no period of residence that will *certainly* exempt one from it, and the cemetery records show the fact that people sometimes die of yellow fever after having been here five, ten, or more years. Residence, then, does not prove it, for people die of other fevers, and all the class of zymotic diseases, after two, three, five, ten, and more years. Hence there is no immunity from death from fevers, and the nearest approach to it here, as elsewhere, is to be derived from the correctness of individual habits, and particularly in relation to temperance. It is unquestionably the result of experience, that these habits have a more injurious influence in this climate than farther north. This important truth is only in accordance with the characteristics of all warm climates, where it is universally acknowledged that such habits almost uniformly abbreviate life, by acting in a line with all the injurious influences of such climate; accordingly, perhaps the most temperate people are to be found in warm climates.

All large cities are mainly aided by accessions of population from extraneous sources; to attempt, then, to separate this population, which in many American towns is so very large, would be, firstly, an impossible thing, and secondly, would be of little comparative avail, if accomplished. Although a large proportion of the mortality may be derived from the recent arrivals, yet he who has frequently examined and studied the Cemetery reports, (as every man who pretends to a desire to reach the truth should,) will be satisfied, that a large proportion of the mortality is also derived, not only from the natives, but from those whose residence here has been five, ten, twenty, thirty and forty years; but whether they have been here a longer or a shorter period is really of very little importance — the character for salubrity must be derived from the fact of their living or dying: now whether this takes place during what some are pleased to term the 'acclimating process, or period,' is of very little consequence; the stamp of vitativeness is what is desired, and the real question is — whether the chance of living in this city is as good as it is elsewhere in the ordinary fluctuating condition of the population, which characterises all American cities at least, and if not, what can be done to make it so, and what are the remedies to be applied?

The only application I propose to make of this remark is, that, with the extension of our improvements, the climate is becoming ameliorated, and that when, by the application of science and skill in completing the alterations in our physical condition, which can easily be accomplished, and the climate shall become fixed and stationary, my impression is, that the bugbear of yellow fever will have disappeared from among us. This is not only not unreasonable, but in accordance with all experience in various parts of our own country, where this formidable disease has been finally shut out by sanitary regulations. Passing from this, with which you are all familiar, I will mention some that are still more striking from abroad. England was in the seventeenth century desolated by plagues; it has disappeared under the influence of these very regulations. Such, too, has been the fact in the greater part of Europe, where (in many parts of it) the average duration of life, up to the times we live in, has nearly doubled from the same cause. But I pass over these and nearly all the cities to the north and east of us in our own country, where it has been put to defiance by the strictness of their police regulations, to invite your attention to a country and climate in so many respects identical with our own, that I am sure it will be both striking and interesting,—I mean Egypt. The plague (which to that country is what the yellow fever is to this) exists in a sporadic form every year, and the epidemic form about every ten years, and where during a recent outbreak (in 1835) it was fatal to upwards of 66 per cent. of its inhabitants! nay, I may say, *natives*, consisting of Negroes, Malays and Arabs. I gave in a note to a preceding page the relative mortality, the difference falling upon the populations in close proportion to *their general sanitary condition*. The mortality was least among those Europeans who live in airy well-conditioned houses, and severest on those who live in the most crowded and filthiest manner. If we consult history, we shall find, that during the reign of the last of the Pharaohs,—during the 194 years of the occupation of Egypt by the Persians,—the 301 years during the dominion of Alexander,—the dynasty of the Ptolemies and a great portion of that of Rome, EGYPT WAS FREE FROM PLAGUE! This absence of any epidemic for the long space of time during which good administration and the sanitary police of the country conquered the producing causes of this most formidable malady, justifies the expectation that the same appliances will be followed by the same results here.* This should be very solacing to us, and should arouse and direct those energies, of which we have more than any other people on the face of the earth, and for the best reason, we are the actual beneficiaries of them, to adopt such remedies as will speedily correct the mortality now existing, and furnish the blessings of health to the finest country in America.

In elucidation of this great subject, let me now invite the attention of the Society particularly to the coincidence, if not

---

* See report of General Board of Health of England.

the connection of the great physical changes, noted in table D, with the salubrity. Thus, we had the first advent of yellow fever during the digging of the canal Carondelet, in 1794–'97. There was a great crevasse in 1816, and extensive paving in 1817—previous to the great fevers of 1817, '19;—extensive pavements in 1824, and up to 1832. The average mortality then was, you see, very great—more than five per cent. In 1830, a violent storm drove the waters of the lake up to Dauphin-street. In 1832–'5, we dug the great canal of the Bank, costing the lives of some 6 or 7000 of its laborers: what effect it had on the two great epidemics of cholera and yellow fever of 1832–'3, I leave it for you to judge. In 1836, the draining machine drained the large section below the canal Carondelet, and in 1835–'9, the forest growth was removed. We had epidemics in 1837, '9, '41: during 1845–'50 the important section betwen the two canals just in the rear of the heart of the city was cleared, and the immense canals dug and the whole drained; and the crevasse of 1849 extended the inundation of the river as far in the centre of the city as Carondelet-street. What influence they had on the disastrous mortality of 1847, '8, 9, and '50, of cholera and yellow fever, will not be left in much doubt, after the preceding statements. These coincidences are, at least, very remarkable; but that they have connection, seems to be in accordance with all experience of the effect of first disturbing the virgin soil of a country, and laying it bare to the influences of an almost tropical sun; of which examples enough might be adduced. These valuable statistical facts will also convince you of the propriety of making, *at once*, all those alterations and improvements in our physical condition upon which our future salubrity so much depends, and that they should be made during the winter season,* to which little attention, I believe, has been paid heretofore. But that all these improvements will finally restore salubrity to the city, is demonstrable *a priori*, from all that has occurred, not only in our own country, but abroad.

I have heretofore limited myself pretty much to the suburbs and neighborhood of the city, and to general causes showing con-

---

* See, in Chart No. I., the line of relative mortality of each month in the year.

ditions that have been most disastrous to the health of the place: let us approach a little nearer, and enter the city itself, and see if we cannot discover conditions deeply affecting its salubrity, and which would be highly injurious even in the latitude of fifty, much less at thirty.

The population of New Orleans and Lafayette, by the recent census, amounts to about 130,000, being near 18,000 to the square mile, showing by the census returns 6.16 to each house, with an average annual temperature of about 67°.

Let us see, then, to what the insalubrity of our city is mainly indebted. It is impaired by—

1st, Bad air;
2d, Privies, Cemeteries, various manufactories, stables, slaughter houses, etc.;
3d, Bad water—stagnant water;
4th, Bad habits;
5th, Bad milk.

It is quite out of the question that I should, in the compass of a single report, (already too much prolonged), go into detail in the examination of each of these and many other causes, by which the salubrity of New Orleans is impaired. I leave these, then, to where they most properly belong—to the special reports of your vigilant Board of Health, (where they have already attracted much notice), and proceed to consider into what they are resolvable, etc.

I. and II. *Bad air*, etc. The greatest sources of *impurity of air* arise from privies, the offal from kitchens, stables, stores, markets, streets, manufactories, etc.

It is estimated that a population of 130,000 produces annually 5633 tons of night soil, and 43,000 tons of urine: these may be doubled from domestic animals, and from other sources are at least as much more; making the frightful aggregate of about 150,000 tons, (including more than 3000 dead bodies buried in the Cemeteries in *the city limits*), of organic matter submitted to the putrefactive fermentation every year, under our very noses, on an area of $7\frac{1}{4}$ square miles! It is in vain to say that the night soil is removed to the river, urine sunk into the soil, and the offals carried a mile or two in the rear, and bodies buried in vaults: all are long enough exposed to contaminate the atmosphere, and those buried are constantly impairing the purity of the air we breathe, and poisoning the water we daily drink.

III. Bad water is probably more injurious to health than bad air, as it acts far more rapidly when taken into the stomach than when taken into the lungs, for venous absorption admits of no selection; it is taken immediately into the lungs and circulated through the system, and as water is capable of holding in solution a greater quantity of foreign matter than air, it is more concentrated. Professor Hoffman has stated that 1000 gallons of water will dissolve 25 gallons of nitrogen, 6 gallons of oxygen, 1000 gallons of carbonic acid, 50,000 gallons of ammonia — the very gas which escapes so largely from privies and the police filth of every dirty town, carrying with it vegetable and animal matters in a high state of putrescency. Hence it is, that our cisterns, and particularly when near the privies, (*as they usually are!*) are sure to be contaminated thereby, and, indeed, every source of filth in its neighborhood.*

It must be highly gratifying to every intelligent mind to be enabled here to apply the facts derived from the deductions of science in the true explanation of this vitally-important subject. You will agree with me, I am sure, in the belief that the utility of science is to be estimated from its capacity to be applied to the practical purposes of life — advancing our comforts and heightening our enjoyments. We have this beautifully exemplified in the important fact stated in the former part of this report (and other and abundant evidences could be furnished) of the connection of a *still atmosphere with disease, and both with a high dew-point*. This presses on us, with all its force, the necessity of ventilation, and it becomes doubly important when with the *damp, still air* of our backyards, the accumulation of

---

* Since the delivery of this report, several who heard it have had their attention called to the subject, and consulted me in relation to sources of impurity of the water in their cisterns, from some cause to them unknown. On examination, it was satisfactorily ascertained that in several instances it was most palpably attributable to the vicinage of their privies — in others, to coal containing much sulphur, etc.

the concentrated filth of a family, including the privy and kitchen offal, in the direct neighborhood of that which is of the last importance to keep pure, viz., the water we drink and use for all domestic wants. Then comes the additionally important fact, derived from science, (mentioned bfore,) that all the noxious gases given off above by these excrementitious remains are absorbed, with destructive rapidity, by this very water! Thus the force and value of the highly satisfactory explanation becomes too apparent to be questioned, and too important to be overlooked.

IV. It is impossible to overlook the effects of intemperance, especially in a warm climate; probably no cause is so effective in undermining the constitution, impairing the *vis-vitæ*, and increasing the liability to disease, as it. There is no disease it does not aggravate; there is no constitution it benefits. The most cursory examination of our cemetery reports of the causes of death will satisfy any professional man, at least, how vast have been the additions to it from an undue indulgence in this vicious habit, and especially of all that large class which gives so baleful a reputation to this climate, I mean the zymotic.* To show the effect of habits upon health in this climate, I have constructed Chart III. to illustrate the different mortalities of males and females. Chart II. (exhibiting the different mortalities between blacks and whites) will show the same to a certain extent, for we find it to be to our *interest to keep our slaves, at least, temperate;* but it was particularly intended to exhibit the different influences of the climate upon the two races.

V. *Bad Milk.*— The mortality in the city of New Orleans of all under five years of age is upwards of 30 per cent., notwithstanding the proverbial kindliness of the climate to our young population, and the mildness of most of the diseases to which they are everywhere subject, such as cholera-infantum, whooping-cough, croup, etc., which, in the northern cities, takes

---

* To my unprofessional readers I may say, that this class particularly embraces endemic and epidemic diseases, as fevers, cholera, dysentery, diarrhœa, etc.

off more than 50 per cent., and in New York, 55 per cent. of all under that age! This immense mortality has been ascribed, nay, almost demonstrated, to arise, with every reasonable probability, to BAD MILK. That the same cause exists here, to some extent, there is no doubt.

Now, the great and important practical question, to which all else is subsidiary, occurs, CAN ALL THIS BE REMEDIED? Are we suffering from 'medicable ills'? or must a mortality of more than $5\frac{1}{2}$ per cent. be suffered to continue — the city to remain slowly to increase, be stationary, or decline under the great rivalry of other more favored spots? as the rapid improvements of science can almost every where supply the almost unequalled advantages here offered to us by nature. Every intelligent physician will at once join in the impulsive response of every Louisianian, *that there must be remedies*, and that WE MUST APPLY THEM.

Let us see what they are:

The great object is to remove filth of all kinds as soon as possible, before it contaminates the air we breathe and the water we drink and cook with, and use for all domestic purposes. This is done by SEWERS, and there is no city in the world better adapted to them,—where the power to answer their purposes is to be had, as it were, without expense, and where they would do a tythe as much good as they would here. I have no time to go into details now; the demonstration has, I must hope, been made in the Board of Health Report of 1849, together with the plan, drawing, etc. It is not to be doubted that *all the filth* that contaminates the atmosphere, from which we have anything to fear, can thus be made away with, and that speedily:—night-soil, urine, kitchen and street filth, etc., all, indeed, excepting the dead, and the few cemeteries within the limits of the corporation should be immediately closed, and all slaughter-houses, manufactories and extensive stables, removed to the outskirts.

All present privies, below or in the soil, should be immediately *emptied and filled up*, and, in their places, jars or barrels, impermeable to fluids or gases, substituted for them, with proper valvular coverings to prevent the escape of gases.* At present, the water is so near the surface, except in and near Levee-street, that no great depth can be excavated but the water rises in it near the surface, and, in rainy seasons, it is subject to overflow; and as we know that night-soil floats on water, *it is always* near the surface, and gives off its noxious gases to contaminate the atmosphere. The members of the Board of Health full well know the trouble our health wardens have every year, during the rainy season, (which occurs at mid-summer,) to remove the constant complaints made to us upon this subject. My impression is, that here is our only remedy, — *no under-ground privies;* and it will recommend itself by its great economy, as well as for its cleanliness and salubrity.

All the present draining-canals about the city should be covered, as the Melpomene, Gormley, Claiborne, and those going to the basins of the draining companies; low lots filled up, and all stagnant water prevented, for in this condition evaporation concentrates its poisons—vegetable infusoriæ, of the class called algæ, as well as fungoid vegetation, are rapidly generated. Many tribes of these vegetable productions appear to die with great rapidity—sometimes in one or two days—and then decompose. Immediately after these, animalcular life appears. Stagnant water is the most favorable to this order of vegetable productions, which, in giving rise to animalcular life, appears to keep pace with the animalised excreta discharged in the house-drainage of towns. Certain degrees of motion in water are unfavorable to the production of algæ and other infusorial plants, the tissues of which are destroyed by brisk motion.† The same round of life and death also takes place in open and shallow reservoirs, and in open cisterns where the water is frequently changed. The eminent German naturalist, Ehrenberg, as one result of very extended observations, established the fact that the existence of visible animalculæ generally indicates the pre-

---

* Since the delivery of this report, I understand there is a depot for, and a manufacturer of, an apparatus of this kind, in Exchange-alley, near the St. Louis Ho'el.

† It has been demonstrated here that the filthy water of our gutters, by brisk motion, in the short space of a half-a-dozen squares, becomes much purified.

sence of a lower series of invisible animalculæ, descending in magnitude to the smallest monad of the most simple structure— so small, that there is probably no smaller organized creature on which it can feed, while, as is commonly conceived, by arresting organised matter on the very limits of the organic world, and converting it into its own nutriment, it furnishes, in its turn, sustenance to higher orders of animalcular life. Be this as it may, it is very certain that the presence of animalculæ in large numbers indicates the existence of animal and vegetable matter, usually in a state of decomposition, which invariably acts injuriously if the water containing them is used largely for purposes of food, and the effects may be more immediate and marked when the animalculæ are large and numerous.*

Light is also necessary for the production of infusoria and fungoid vegetation, and their formation is prevented by such covering as excludes the light and heat of the sun.

In an alluvion soil like ours, the most perfect paving is that which entirely excludes the possibility of evaporation from the subsoil, and that is by stone blocks united by cement with an angle of inclination to the side gutters, and these to the sewers. Running water from the river or water-works should be in constant use in dry weather in summer, and at such other times as may be ordered by the Board of Health: every street and yard should be cleared *every day, and the filth at once removed.* Health wardens should be appointed for every few squares, whose duty should be to inspect every yard and court *every day,* and every privy weekly or monthly. Trees should be planted in the streets to absorb the noxious gases and give out those which refresh and purify the atmosphere — to moderate the influence of reflected heat from brick walls and houses. It is a law of nature, that the vegetable and animal kingdoms should be, as it were, supplemental the one to the other: animals by breathing and exhaling air, load it with carbonic acid, and render it noxious to themselves; while vegetables absorb the acid gas, and give out oxygen in its stead, and thus supply the animal kingdom with vital air. Then again, whatever elements an animal takes from

---

* Vide Report of the General Board of Health of England.

the soil as food, it returns again to the earth in a different form, noxious to itself, but nevertheless furnishing to the vegetable kingdom abundant and wholesome nourishment. It is thus that the organic elements complete their circuit in living beings. Nothing is lost; it is only reproduced in another form. These principles lie at the root of the whole science of agriculture; while they constitute the basis of all economical and sanitary arrangements.*

It has been said by very high authority, Dr. Jarvis, that wherever differences of vitality are found to exist in connection with differences of circumstances, condition, locality, or manner of life, it may be assumed as probable, at least, if not certain, that the former are the consequences of the latter. It is an unquestionable principle, that in the operations of life, as well as in those of dead matter, there is no event without a cause adequate to produce it.

It is equally certain, that in life as well as in death, in similar circumstances and conditions, like causes produce like results. In this law of vital action, there is no uncertainty or invariableness. There is no more caprice or mystery in the ebb or flow of life,—in the maintenance of health, in the cause of sickness, or in the event of death, than in the flow and ebb of the tides, in the movement of the stars, or in the action of gravitation.

It must be admitted as an universal fact, that from any definite amount of vitalizing or destructive influence acting upon living beings, there will follow a definite and corresponding amount of health, strength and life, or of sickness, weakness and death. Between the amount of the cause and the amount of the effect there is an exact relation. No matter how weak or how powerful may be the deteriorating cause, precisely corresponding to that will be the deterioration.' It is thus demonstrable and demonstrated, if we ever expect or wish a healthy city, we must remove the known and well-ascertained causes of its insalubrity, and fortunately for us there is no difficulty about it which cannot be removed or surmounted, by determination, enterprise, science and capital. The health of a place is an indispensable element

---

* Vide 'Liverpool Health of Towns' Advocate.'

in its prosperity; nothing can be permanent, without this greatest of blessings; and *whatever the cost*, in the end it will be *cheap*, if this shall be the result. The true wealth of a country consists in its people, and particularly at the productive age; of this age, Louisiana, and particularly New Orleans, has a large proportion: it is not only larger than any portion of the United States, but of any part of the world. The Chart No. III. I now again advert to, as well as all our Cemetery reports, to show that this, too, is the age of death here, and that the period is the autumn, and particularly September.* In a sickly country, not only two or more are constantly sick and withdrawn from the active duties of life, with all its attendant expenses, for every one that dies, (and, indeed, it is estimated, that there are actually twenty cases of sickness to one of death), but more, there is a half sickly valetudinarian existence, which materially trenches upon and consumes valuable time. Besides all this, a sickly country is the main cause of that absenteeism which not only deprives the State of the services of a large portion of her citizens, but abstracts from profitable use and investment at home, millions of her natural resources; retards the advancement of the permanent population of the city; keeps down the value of city property, and prevents all those social and literary enjoyments, and those extensive beneficences which a concentrated healthy population always gives rise to, and enhances and secures

From the foregoing observations, several important facts are made perfectly clear to the mind of the reporter: First, that a large mortality has existed in this city for a long series of years, and particularly during the periods when the great physical changes have been made; second, that these causes are well known and perfectly removeable; third, with prudent habits, acclimation — if such a thing exists at all now, specifically, of which there is great doubt — is no longer to be dreaded; and it is satisfactorily shown that the yellow fever is departing from among us; and, finally, that with this difficulty removed, we have as fine a climate as any in America;—and that this is

---

* See also Chart No. I.—the mortuary line.

proved, not only from the strictest and most extensive meteorological observations; but from the remarkable salubrity enjoyed in the rural districts of the vicinity. To this I need add but one remark,— that, as our duties result from our relations — to the city— to ourselves— to society, (and it is utterly impossible to waive or alienate them,) every consideration of self-interest, of health, enjoyment and prosperity, as well as the warning voice of past pestilences, with the hope and the prospect of securing a comparative stationary condition, on the finest theatre in the world for advancement, while every city is outstripping us in the career of prosperous fortune, urge us to make the improvements required. The single fact—the basis of so many others—is, that capitalists, proverbially timid, will not invest permanently where the mortality is double what it is elsewhere; and you cannot expect an increase of a stationary population of that middle class, mechanics, manufacturers, laborers, and others — the bone and sinew of the land —where there is not as fair an average of health, as can elsewhere be procured in our country.

But I must close. I have trespassed too long on your indulgence, but I cannot permit this opportunity to pass without again referring to the peculiar position in which our city is placed, even at the expense of some repetition: in sight, as it were, of the promised land, with the golden fruit ready to be plucked, we wilfully neglect the important subject of our sanitary relations, and thus prevent the fulfilment of our manifest destiny. I have bestowed much trouble on the important facts I have given you, presuming that the elucidation of the truth with regard to our actual condition will be the means of its correction. The time is truly passed in this enlightened age, when assertion will be taken for fact, and that an intelligent people can be long mystified by statements, however high their source. That many —nay, most of us—have been led to entertain erroneous impressions with regard to our sanitary condition, for a long series of years, is unquestionable. We have been so misled by *false* OFFICIAL STATEMENTS, from the highest sources*, which have

* United States census of 1840.

lulled us into a fatal security, superseded, in some measure, investigation into our actual condition, and thus prevented those corrective measures indispensable to our safety.

This excuse exists no longer; we now *know sufficient of our condition* to be convinced that vast improvements are required; and it would be a poor compliment to pay to an enlightened and wealthy community, as this is, to say that it will hesitate one moment to apply the proper remedy. I see a full guarantee of this promise in the newly-awakened interest this subject is assuming among us. When the curiosity of this public is fully aroused, it will only be satisfied with the truth. This truth is a truly painful one, but it is with as much pride as pleasure I venture the statement, corroborated by the laborious investigation of many years, that the *condition is a removeable one;* and that, by the application of science and skill to enterprise and industry, perseveringly pursued, all can be accomplished that the most sanguine could anticipate, or the most enthusiastic desire. No medical man of reputation would venture the assertion that our condition cannot be vastly ameliorated: the physical aspects of nature are as much, if not more susceptible of improvement for the sanitary condition, than for the enterprises of commerce. In the great competition for supremacy for the western trade, we do not start even in the race unless we are upon a par with them in a sanitary point of view. With all right in this, the game is in our own hands, and it is all comprehended in a few words,—sewerage, and a proper system of policeing. The meteorological tables will show you we have the ideal temperature for the most perfect health and enjoyment, with an almost entire freedom from those extremes which are so injurious to health farther north. It is true we have too much moisture, but then the improvements suggested would, if carried into effect, in a great measure remove this excess. With the adoption of these improvements as a basis, all else will soon follow, for, with health, a permanent population, wealth, taste, refinement will soon develop our delightful climate, and we shall be in the uninterrupted enjoyment of the most pleasant residence in America.

I trust, under your auspices, the public will be invited to take an interest in the important connection of experimental science with practical, every-day facts, as shown, for instance, in the elucidation made by the hygrometer of the necessity of ventilation in this climate, in the condition which exists in the *still air* of most of our back yards, and too many of our houses, with what has been shown of its actual condition in a *calm atmosphere* in other situations;—of the connection of this atmosphere with moisture, and of moisture with disease. This has been most satisfactorily shown in Table B, of the hygrometry of the winds, of which various illustrations are given;—of the facility with which the water we drink and use for all culinary purposes becomes contaminated by being placed, by a singular perversion of good taste, in juxtaposition with all the filth of the family! I again call your attention, too, to the interesting statement in the text, first pointed out by a French meteorologist, of the discovery of the actual *means* of daily temperatures when certain plants (enumerated) would flower (and by implication, as it is a law of all plants); and in our country, where it has been shown of the return of great epidemic visitations, on the occurrence of certain meteorological conditions, known antecedent to their outbreak. The same principles applied to the cultivation of our great staples—sugar-cane and cotton—will announce to us, at the periods of their first maturation, (the flowering of the one and the ripening of the other,) the probable produce from each during that season, barring accidents; and, being the results of actual numerical calculation, will prevent that uncertainty, and of course put an end to that speculation, so ruinous to the producer.

These views alone, demonstrate the importance of keeping accurate meteorological records of our condition, not only for health, but for agriculture and commerce. Had the facts which these principles explain been known to our intelligent and enterprising planters, the products of our great staples would long since have been extended all over the State, and been much more certain crops than they now are. They mostly confine themselves, at present, to the very slow and expensive one of empirical experiments, instead of applying principles at once, and boldly dashing forward wherever they are applicable, with all the assurance of success which comes of scientific deduction. An illustration is furnished of this in the very recent cultivation of the cane in the Red river district, and the highlands of our State, where it is cultivated with as much success, if not more, than in the lower river districts to which it had been so long restricted, while it may as well have been cultivated in the others twenty years earlier!

But, gentlemen, there is another fact which claims your very special attention: No country of any importance is so shamefully destitute of records of the past, and particularly of mortuary records, as this.

You would deem me very extravagant if I should inform you how much I think your interest has been sacrificed by this disgraceful neglect. With the finest climate, soil and position in our country, you are kept *half a century back* of what you would have been had the facts been known, by a proper registry-law of your births, deaths, and marriages, and a meteorological record of this and various parts of your State;—the one thoroughly to record what the climate is, and the other to exhibit the effects of that climate—each bearing upon the other. When the climate or condition of a place is found to be inimical to the health of its inhabitants, it must be attributable to certain causes, which should always lead to an examination. Experimental investigations, under the direction of science, are then employed to find them out, and when so discovered, there is little difficulty in removing them. I will give you a very striking instance: Some years ago, the people of Liverpool were in the habit of boasting of their health,—*as we are in the habit of doing.* The facts developed through the admirable registry-law of England, soon showed that they were suffering under the disastrous mortality of about 1 in 19, or 5.26 per cent.! They soon took the alarm; and, on examination, the cause was found palpably to arise mainly from their extensive, filthy cellar population. This was immediately abated, and their salubrity was soon increased to 1 in 27, or 3.70 per cent.! The following pages will show a much larger mortality here: but the heart of every patriot and philanthropist among us may yet throb with delight, when, through a similar appliance, we shall be blessed with similar ameliorations.

From what has been before said, but necessarily alluded to very briefly, it is in the power of sanitary measures to accomplish almost everything we could desire. Those who have most fully investigated this subject, admit that by these means we can procure a state of health where the mortality does not exceed 2 per cent. Then cast your eyes over Table D, and you will see, through our neglect and ignorance—and, of course, the former resulting from the latter—we have actually had a mortality, during more than sixty years, on an average, of nearly twice and a half as much as that! and during some series of years near three and a half times as much! while, in some single years, it has exceeded *four times* as much, or 8.33 per cent.! though there are years in the group, as in 1812, when the mortality was only 2.22 per cent., and in 1827, when it was only 2.25. These are highly important facts to be remembered. They show that the former mortality does not so much belong to our position, AS ITS ABUSE; and it belongs to this intelligent public to determine *whether it shall be continued*, for it is hoped that it has been satisfactorily demonstrated in this report that it is entirely in our power to remove them. The longer continuance of such a state of things is not only ruinous to the best interests of the city, but a reproach to the age we live in, if, by any means, they can be remedied.

In taking leave of this most important and interesting topic, I must express the hope I have that you will take a manly share in considering its bearing upon our sanitary state, and our future prosperity, and come with a free and strong help to its accomplishment. There is a mighty incubus that is paralysing the slumbering energies of this great community; and, with the long delusion we have labored under, it requires no ordinary moral courage to express the thorough conviction I entertain, sustained by the facts in this paper, that it arises mainly from the sanitary condition, in defiance of the boastings and taunts of those who draw their facts from their fancies, and construct their opinions upon their wishes. An average mortality of 5.83 per cent., or 1 in 17-70, for the last ten years, is rather a too serious matter for the city fathers to contemplate or set quiet under, while the remedies are in reach, and while they hold the power to apply them. Figures are stubborn things, for they are facts; the imagination quails under their influence; and all reasoning upon such topics without them, or against them, having nothing to rest upon, must fall to the ground.

The glaring fact of our almost stationary condition, in this AGE OF PROGRESS, stares us in the face. Enterprise is abroad. Vigorous competition is putting every place, whose position is far inferior to ours, naturally, ahead of us. The main responsibility rests, first, upon those who represent the city in the councils, to take the initiative, to which they have been repeatedly urged by the Board of Health, to adopt such a system of sanitary reform as will remove the greatest obstacles to our advancement. The future welfare of New Orleans depends upon their enlightened and zealous efforts for the public good. They cannot evade it, if they would. They have an OFFCIAL CONSULTATIVE Board* with whom to divide responsibility, who will cheerfully aid them in their important duties. A *longer postponement is a sacrifice of an important public duty.* Alone, I might shrink from the freedom I have taken with your actions and opinions; but, gentlemen, with the aid and sanction of the intelligent and scientific body I see before me, proper representatives of the enlightened sentiment of the profession in all parts of the State, I feel I am but the organ of your views. Though I will not presume to assert that you endorse all the opinions I have expressed in this report, yet, as the main facts are undeniable, and the deductions from them obvious and fair, I shall at least take it for granted that you so far concur with me that you join in the call for a thorough scrutiny into the facts, and, if they are sustained by the proofs, you will aid in the adoption of suitable measures to remove the causes of disease, and improve and promote the public health.

---

* Board of Health.

TABLE A.

AVERAGE MONTHLY HYGROMETRICAL CONDITION OF NEW ORLEANS,

At different periods of the day, for Eight Years.

	Dew-Point, Average,			Hygrometric Scale. Amount of Moisture, Average, (Saturation being 1000,)			Elasticity of Vapor, Average,			Weight of Vapor in a cubic foot, in grains, Average,			Degree of Dryness on the Thermometric Scale, Average,		
	AT Sunrise.	AT Midday.	AT 9 P.M.	AT Sunrise	AT Midday	AT 9 P.M	AT Sunrise	AT Midday	AT 9 P.M	AT Sunrise.	AT Midday.	AT 9 P.M.	AT Sunrise.	AT Midday.	AT 9 P.M.
January	0°.97	51°.71	53°.86	.878	.724	.876	.414	.442	.490	4.663	4.889	5.445	4°.05	9°.40	4.07
February	43.59	50.86	45.06	.822	.636	.714	.319	.408	.340	3.658	4.483	3.700	5.88	13.66	10.00
March	58.00	58.57	56.08	.863	.678	.731	.511	.542	.492	5.667	5.933	5.425	4.26	14.09	7.93
April	59.46	67.06	61.67	.957	.695	.803	.551	.673	.588	6.102	7.453	6.432	2.54	13.59	6.83
May	65.48	66.50	67.72	.919	.661	.844	.667	.719	.716	7.212	7.638	7.757	2.75	13.08	5.51
June	71.38	73.95	73.16	.937	.718	.852	.827	.868	.853	8.934	9.260	9.158	2.70	10.46	4.87
July	76.24	75.42	75.50	.970	.767	.890	.910	.931	.936	10.161	9.564	9.962	1.56	8.69	3.73
August	75.85	75.59	77.06	.956	.739	.879	.931	.918	.968	10.039	9.601	10.336	1.77	9.82	4.18
September	70.61	73.68	73.66	.909	.746	.792	.798	.867	.808	8.637	9.216	9.46	2.70	9.95	7.14
October	60.39	62.73	61.80	.892	.707	.833	.562	.611	.590	6.201	6.488	6.550	3.91	12.26½	5.95
November	50.17	54.27	55.87	.839	.651	.842	.442	.453	.496	4.881	5.005	5.534	5.36	12.56	5.87
December	51.15	52.43	51.97	.914	.719	.856	.389	.420	.429	4.941	4.530	5.374	2.08	9.52	4.55
TOTALS, {Annual average.}	61.16	63.56	62.95	.905	.703	8.26	.610	.654	.647	6.758	7.007	6.678	3.30	11.42	5.89

[48]

TABLE B.
HYGROMETRY OF EACH OF THE PRINCIPAL WINDS AT NEW ORLEANS, AND WHEN CALM.

DEGREE OF DRYING POWER.			AMOUNT OF MOISTURE. [Saturation being 1000.]			ELASTICITY OF THE VAPOR.			WEIGHT OF VAPOR IN A CUBIC FOOT, *In grains.*		
1st	N.W.	11°.29	1st	N.W.	.677	1st	N.W.	.468	1st	N.W.	5.136
2d	N.	10 .06	2d	N.	.698	2d	N.	.534	2d	N.	5.819
3d	S.W.	10 .03	3d	S.W.	.727	3d	N.E.	.630	3d	N.E.	6.847
4th	W.	10 .01	4th	W.	.740	4th	W.	.646	4th	W.	6.915
5th	N.E.	9 .28	5th	S.	.761	5th	E.	.646	5th	S.	7.181
6th	E.	8 .84	6th	N.E.	.763	6th	S.W.	.664	6th	E.	7.213
7th	S.	8 .21	7th	E.	.768	7th	S.	.743	7th	S.W.	7.229
8th	S.E.	7 .56	8th	S.E.	.720	8th	S.E.	.759	8th	S.E.	8.030
9th	CALM	5 .17	9th	CALM.	.929	9th	CALM.	.761	9th	CALM.	8.254

N. B.— To my scientific readers I observe that some few small errors in the above could only have been ascertained when the *results* were arrived at — but at too late a period to re-calculate sixty pages of figures.

TABLE C.
STATEMENT OF THE WINDS IN NEW ORLEANS — BY MONTHS AND SEASONS.

	N.	N.E.	E.	S.E.	S.	S.W	W.	N.W	Calm.	Explanation.
January	4.¼	4.¼	5.	3.¼	3.¼	1.¾	2.	2.¼	0.½	
February	4.¼	3.½	4.¾	2.¾	3.	2.½	1.¼	4.	0.¼	
March	4.½	2.¾	5.½	3.¼	7.	2.½	1.½	2.½	0.¼	
April	1.½	2.¾	6.¼	4.¾	6.¾	2.½	2.¾	2.	0.¼	
May	2.¾	2.¾	5.½	4.	6.¾	3.¾	1.½	2.¼	1.	
June	1.¾	1.¾	6.¼	4.½	4.¾	6.	1.¾	1.¼	1.	Being on an average of 11 years — 1835–'42 and '48–'50.
July	1.	2.	5.	5.	6.	4.	3.	1.½	3.	
August	3.½	3.½	4.	3.½	4.½	4.	3.¼	1.¾	2.	
September	6.	6.½	6.¼	1.¾	2.¼	1.½	1.¾	1.¾	0.¾	
October	6.¼	5.¼	7.	1.½	1.¾	1.	2.	3.	1.	
November	5.¾	1.	4.¾	3.¼	3.¼	1.	1.	3.¼	0.¼	
December	7.¼	4.¼	5.½	3.	3.	1.¾	1.¾	1.¾	1.¼	

BY SEASONS.

Winter	16.	11.¾	15.¼	9.	9.¼	6.	5.	8.¼	2.	
Spring	8.½	8.¼	17.¼	12.	20.¼	8.¾	5.½	6.¾	1.¾	Total number of days' wind each season.
Summer	6.¼	7.¼	15.¼	13.	15.¼	14.	8.	4.¾	6.	
Autumn	18.¼	12.¾	18.	6.¼	7.¼	3.¼	4.¾	8.¼	2.¼	

Winter	1st	3d	2d	5th	4th	7th	8th	6th	9th	
Spring	5th	6th	2d	3d	1st	4th	8th	7th	9th	Relative frequency of each wind during each season.
Summer	7th	6th	1st	4th	2d	3d	5th	8th	9th	
Autumn	1st	3d	2d	6th	5th	8th	7th	4th	9th	

BY THE YEAR.

3d	5th	1st	4th	2d	6th	8th	7th	9th	Relative frequency of each wind during the year.
49.	40.	66.½	40.¾	52.½	32.¼	23.¼	27.¾	12.¼	

TABLE D.

Exhibiting the Mortality of the city of New Orleans since 1787, (with exceptions as stated,) with the ratios, the relative proportion dying at the Charity Hospital, and the dates of great physical changes in and about the city.

YEARS EMBRACED.	AVERAGE POPULATION.	AVERAGE MORTALITY.	RATIO 1 to —	RATIO PER CENT	AVERAGE CHARITY HOSPITAL MORTALITY TO CITY MORTALITY. PER CENT.	DATES OF PHYSICAL ALTERATIONS AND IMPROVEMENTS IN CITY AND NEIGHBORHOOD.
10 years, 1787–'97.	7,020	.488	14.38	6.95	- -	1785, '91, '99.—Crevasses above, affecting the city. 1796.—Fortifications made around the city, and surrounded by trenches.
6 years, 1811–'15.	28,741	.989	30.82	3.42	- -	1794-'97.—Canal Carondelet dug.
1816–'20.	37,985	1.517	29.15	3.95	17.77	1811.—Canal Carondelet cleaned out. 1816.—Crevasse. 1817.—First Pavements commenced. 1820.—Wooden side-walks, and curbing removed and replaced with stone. 1817–'20.—Large enclosures of the batture.†
*4 years, omitting 1821. 1821–'25.	44,539	2.085	21.17	4.72	17.60	1824.—Gormley's Canal and Basin dug, about 1824–'22. 1824–'32.—Extensive paving done.
1826–'30.	47,834	1.707	27.68	3.61	21.82	1825–'28.—Melpomene Canal adopted from a natural drain, cleaned out and deepened.
*4 years, omitting 1832. 1831–'35.	58,570	3.503	18.22	5.92	27.11	1831.—Violent storm inundated back part of the city, to Dauphin street. 1832–'35.—The Bank Canal of the 2d municipality dug to the lake — 7 miles. 1832–'34.—Extensive paving. 1835–'39.—Forest growth cut down in rear of city, first municipality. 1836.—Draining machine on Bayou St. John, drained the section in rear of first municipality.
*4 years, omitting 1837. 1836–'40.	74,262	2.942	25.39	3.96	27.11	1837, October.—Violent storm inundated the rear of the city. Draining company continued their operations.
1841–'45. 1846–'50.	90,000	3.993	23.29	4.48	21.20	1844.—Violent storm inundated the city up to Burgundy street. 1845–'50.—That section of the rear of the city between the canals Carondelet and Bank, in the rear of the central parts of the city, ditched, drained, and forest growth removed.
N.O. and Lafayette, for the last year.	109,693	7.622	15.33	6.93	24.71	1849, May and June.—Extensive inundation from Sauve Crevasse, extending as high up as Carondelet street.
TOTALS...			23.19	4.87	22.38	

* The total mortality of these years could not be procured.
† Extract from the report of the Physico-Medical Society on the epidemic yellow fever of 1820, by Drs. Randolph, Davidson and Marshall: "We would remind the Society of the evident co-existence existing between the enclosure of the batture and the recent unusual consecution of epidemic fevers in this city.

P.S. I intended to have added a column embracing the average annual immigration from abroad; but the record has not been retained at our customhouse anterior to 1845, since when it has averaged about 30,000 per annum; but very few arriving in the summer and fall months.

TABLE E.

STATEMENT of the number of Free and Slave Population, as well as the number of Deaths from Cholera and other Diseases, in the Parishes of the Western District of Louisiana, as taken by the Assistant Marshals, and returned to the United States Marshal's office, under the Census Act of 23d May, 1850.

PARISHES.	INHABITANTS. FREE.	SLAVES.	POPULATION W. District TOTAL.	Mortality FREE. CHOLERA	Mortality SLAVES CHOLERA	TOTAL Cholera, SEPARATED.	TOTAL Mortality	TOTAL MORTALITY PER CENT. WITHOUT CHOLERA.	TOTAL MORTALITY PER CENT. INCLUDING CHOLERA.
Carroll	2,346	6,443	8,789	12	110	122	405	3.22	4.61
Madison	1,418	7,350	8,768	9	138	147	417	3.08	4.75
Tensas	902	8,138	9,040	11	131	142	319	1.96	3.52
Concordia	824	6,934	7,758	3	52	55	171	1.50	2.20
Ouachita	2,300	2,708	5,008	..	..	..	117	....	2.33
Morehouse	1,907	2,006	3,913	8	4	12	260	6.34	6.64
Union	4,778	3,425	8,203	7	4	11	716	8.59	8.72
Jackson	3,407	2,243	5,650	8	4	12	313	5.50	5.53
Catahoula	3,616	3,548	7,164	17	30	47	443	5.52	6.18
Franklin	1,681	1,573	3,254	1	3	4	283	8.58	8.67
Caldwell	1,590	1,232	2,822	2	3	5	185	6.38	6.55
Claiborne	4,949	2,522	7,471	2	4	6	612	8.11	8.19
Bossier	2,507	4,788	7,295	1	19	20	368	4.77	5.05
De Soto	3,566	4,450	8,016	9	9	18	496	5.96	6.18
Caddo	3,667	6,468	10,135	..	..	..	330	....	3.25
Natchitoches	6,345	7,627	13,972	4	15	19	848	5.93	6.06
Sabine	3,347	1,167	4,514	..	6	6	538	11.80	11.91
Rapides*	4,000	9,000	13,000	..	..	..	250	1.49	1.92
Avoyelles	4,166	5,161	9,327	4	26	30	392	3.88	4.20
St. Landry	11,384	10,871	22,255	..	..	..	775	3.29	3.48
Calcasieu	2,957	951	3,908	..	..	..	239	....	6.10
Lafayette	3,560	3,183	6,743	..	..	..	283	....	4.19
Vermillion	2,342	1,067	3,409	1	1	2	218	6.33	6.39
St. Martin	5,198	6,468	11,666	..	..	..	422	3.39	3.61
St. Mary	3,911	9,940	13,851	..	..	..	208	1.44	1.50
Bienville	3,644	1,895	5,539	4	2	6	275	5.04	5.15
Totals	90,312	121,158	211,470	103	561	664	9,883	5.09	5.22

Classification of the Parishes of the Western District of Louisiana:— INCLUDING CHOLERA. EXCLUDING CHOLERA.

1. Ratio of mortality in river parishes, per cent. - - - - - - 3.81   2.46 ⎫ White
2. Do.   do.   in swamp parishes do - - - - - - - 3.52   3.42 ⎬ and
3. Do.   do.   in upland parishes do. - - - - - - 6.21   6.08 ⎭ Colored.

* These numbers are furnished by a correspondent — not published by the Deputy Marshal.

TABLE F.

STATEMENT of the number of DWELLING HOUSES, FREE and SLAVE POPULATION, as well Eastern District of Louisiana, as taken by the different Assistant Marshals, and

	PARISHES.	Number of Dwellings.	INHABITANTS. FREE.	SLAVES.	Population East. District of Louisiana. TOTAL.
1	ORLEANS. *First Municipality—*				
	1st, 2d, and 3d Wards	2154	9,668	1,974	11,642
	4th, 5th, 6th and 7th Wards	3184	23,893	6,136	30,029
	Second Municipality—				
	1st and 2d Wards	1,558	7,676	1,107	8,783
	3d Ward	1,752	9,072	978	10,050
	4th Ward	861	5,680	840	6,520
	5th, 6th and 7th Wards	2,673	23,519	3,162	26,681
	Third Municipality	3,870	19,890	2,812	22,702
	Right bank of Mississippi river	401	2,029	1,057	3,086
2	JEFFERSON				
	1st, 2d, and 3d Wards, Lafayette	2,056	10,929	1,371	12,300
	5th Ward, City of Lafayette, and remainder of Parish	1,769	7,801	4,825	12,626
3	Ascension	755	3,486	7,266	10,752
4	Assumption	926	5,197	5,341	10,538
5	East Feliciana	712	4,084	9,512	13,596
6	West Feliciana	599	2,579	10,666	13,245
7	East Baton Rouge	1044	5,627	6,351	11,978
8	West Baton Rouge	392	1,920	4,351	6,271
9	Iberville	640	3,680	8,607	12,287
10	Lafourche Interior	938	5,166	4,368	9,534
11	Livingston	480	2,543	841	3,384
12	Plaquemine	615	2,611	4,779	7,390
13	Point Coupée	760	3,528	7,812	11,340
14	St. Bernard	283	1,479	2,284	3,763
15	St. Charles	191	988	4,132	5,120
16	St. John the Baptist	530	2,778	4,540	7,318
17	St. James	591	3,317	7,754	11,098
18	St. Tammany	786	4,003	2,363	6,366
19	St. Helen	390	2,366	2,196	4,562
20	Terre Bonne	550	3,396	4,331	7,727
21	Washington	406	2,371	1,037	3,408
	TOTALS	31,266	181,306	122,790	304,096

Mortality of the Country Parishes of Louisiana—Eastern District of La.

	Classification of the Parishes.	Including Cholera. WHITES PER CENT.	COLORED PER CENT.	BOTH, PER CENT.	Excluding Cholera. WHITES PER CENT.	COLORED PER CENT.	BOTH, PER CENT.
1	Ratio of Mortality of the River Parishes, excluding New Orleans, Lafayette and West Feliciana, and including other river towns	2.69	2.45	2.57	1.03	1.42	1.29
2	Ratio of Mortality of the Swamp Parishes	0.63	1.48	1.05	0.44	0.75	0.60
3	Ratio of Mortality of the Upland Parishes	1.74	1.77	1.75	1.57	1.61	1.57

[53]

. . . . TABLE F.

as the number of Deaths from CHOLERA and other Diseases, in the respective Parishes of the returned to the United States Marshal's office, under the Census Act of 23d May, 1850.

Mortality Free Inhabitants.			Mortality Slave Inhabitants.			Ratios of Mortality per cent.			
						WHITES. MORTALITY PER CENT. WITHOUT CHOLERA.	COLORED. MORTALITY PER CENT. WITHOUT CHOLERA.	TOTAL MORTALITY PER CENT. WITHOUT CHOLERA.	TOTAL MORTALITY PER CENT. INCLUDING CHOLERA.
CHOLERA.	OTHER DISEASES.	TOTAL.	CHOLERA.	OTHER DISEASES.	TOTAL.				
22	86	108	19	20	39	0.89	1.01	0.91	1.28
63	281	344	30	58	88	1.18	0.94	1.13	1.43
26	146	172	7	24	31	1.90	2.16	1.94	2.31
51	89	140	6	5	11	0.98	0.51	0.93	1.50
2	11	13	...	1	1	0.20	0.12	0.18	0.21
460	1702	2162	7	22	29	7.24	0.70	6.46	8.24 †
60	302	362	10	71	81	1.52	2.52	1.64	1.95
3	33	36	3	22	25	1.63	2.08	1.78	1.97
52	283	335	8	46	54	2.60	3.36	2.67	3.16
						2.01	1.48	1.96	2.44 *
34	115	149	49	84	133	1.48	1.74	1.58	2.23
3	34	37	81	22	103	0.98	1.11	1.07	1.30
36	41	77	144	59	203	0.79	1.10	0.95	2.66
4	86	90	3	176	179	2.10	1.85	1.93	1.97
13	67	80	18	279	297	2.60	2.62	2.61	2.85
45	101	146	67	98	165	1.79	1.54	1.66	2.60
21	28	49	88	84	172	1.45	1.93	1.78	3.52
14	23	37	143	170	313	0.62	1.97	1.57	2.84
....	...	...	...	9	9	....	0.20	0.10	0.10
5	32	37	5	15	20	1.25	1.78	1.38	1.69
27	56	83	81	83	164	2.14	1.76	1.88	3.34
5	8	13	35	100	135	0.22	1.28	0.95	1.30
...	4	4	9	14	23	0.27	0.61	0.48	0.72
3	12	15	49	61	110	1.21	1.47	1.42	2.44
9	17	26	78	51	129	0.61	1.12	0.93	2.10
5	19	24	89	105	194	0.60	1.15	0.91	1.96
...	58	58	4	41	45	1.45	1.74	1.55	1.62
...	26	26	...	25	25	1.10	1.14	1.12	1.12
2	18	20	7	42	49	0.53	0.97	0.76	0.89
...	23	23	...	6	6	0.97	0.58	0.85	0.85
965	3701	4666	1040	1793	2833	1.05	1.38	1.27	1.90 *

U. S. Marshal's Office,
Eastern District of Louisiana.

New Orleans, April 15, 1850.

WM. P. SCOTT, U. S. M.

By CHAS. A. LABUZAN,

D'y Marshal.

To E. H. BARTON, M.D.

*I have added the per centage of Mortality separately from the cities of New Orleans and Lafayette, as that is done above.
E. H. B

† The Charity Hospital is in this ward, where all the sick emigrants go on their arrival at New Orleans.

EXPLANATION.

In explanation of Tables 'E' and 'F,' it is necessary to state that the deputy marshals, in making their general returns, only specify 'free' and 'slave,' hence the free negroes of the State are classed with the 'white,' and allowance should be made in the mortuary estimates of those tables, until the fiscal digestion of all the specific returns, from Washington. This explanation does not apply to any other portion of the text or the charts, where a contrast is instituted between 'white' and 'colored.'

[*Note to page* 31.]

The true philosophy of what is very loosely called 'acclimation,' is very little understood — the materials do not exist. We know that one latitude, or zone of the earth, is different in what is technically called its 'climate,' from another; that these even differ in their longitudes; that elevation or depression, and the vicinage of mountains, plains or great bodies of water, materially influence it; but farther we cannot go. How difference of soil affects it we know not; that it does affect plants is undeniable; and that even contiguous fields produce different varieties of fruit and other productions; but the cause here is palpable enough — they derive what supports their existence from it, we never do. All we can say, then, positively, and from which to reason, is, that from these positions result a difference of meteorological condition. The exponent, then, of climate, so far as our present positive knowledge extends, is Meteorology. Now, from our ignorance of meteorological conditions, with almost one exception, of different countries, we are limited to the explanation which that one furnishes,—I mean difference of temperature. Let us see, then, what this supplies. The inhabitants of the northern, or cool regions, are generally of the sanguine temperament, with a large development of their sanguiferous and pulmonary systems, with a corresponding power of generating heat, to adapt them to the wants of such a climate. On the contrary, the natives of hot regions have usually the bilious temperament, with the reverse organization, because the requirements of this climate are different, and they get rid of their excess of carbonic acid through other emunctories, and they take in less through their lungs, it not being required, and if it was taken in, they would be over-heated by the combustion it would excite in their systems; hence, then, the predominance of the bilious temperament in hot climates; and it is a matter of observation that temperaments are convertible by long residence — certainly the sanguine becomes bilious through generations,—and in accordance with these principles we find the visitor from the North, of the bilious temperament, is more easily accommodated to the South than he of the sanguine. Dr. Cartwright has clearly shown that the negro requires less pure, or oxygenated, air than the white man, in their much greater adaptation to hot climates. Here, then, is *one positive fact* by which acclimation is explained; and as man is almost the only animal that can adapt himself to different climates, he clearly accomplishes it by the exercise of his intellectual powers in accommodating himself to different temperatures, mainly, by changes in his dress and mode of living; while other animals who survive this change, in a great degree lose the coverings which protected them from northern rigors, on coming to the South. Is there any other *positive, undeniable fact upon the subject?* Habituation to a climate to constitute it — that is, habituation to a certain fixed atmospherical condition, — (and it is owing to our ignorance of the other departments of Meteorology that we are at present compelled to limit it to this) — is, then, but *habituation to a certain range of temperature.* All other explanations are hypothetical — but *petitiones principii,* — and based upon assumptions that are unphilosophical to admit, and I pass them by. The troops transferred by the Pacha of Egypt to the comparatively cold mountains of Greece, from the torrid regions of southern Egypt and Nubia, perished like rotten sheep, without apparent disease. The Laplander, transplanted to Louisiana, would die from excessive heat, if his ordinary power of generating caloric for his indispensable wants, in his cold regions, was not immediately restrained here. Negroes, transferred to colder climates from Africa or the South, suffer great mortality from the change, and particularly from pulmonary disease, from the increased activity required through this system of supplying heat. Monkeys carried to England all die speedily, and mainly of the same disease, if not confined to an atmosphere artificially heated for them; and these illustrations* could be vastly extended in corroboration of the position assumed.

In this view of the subject, acclimation has a wider range and a more specific application, and is not confined to those coming South from the the North. But they are, I believe, unnecessary, for actual experience, *when properly tested,* is against the admission of the absolute necessity of acclimation, to any great extent, from one temperate region to another; at all events, it must be abandoned so far as it depends upon a *fixed physical condition,* as it regards us, for that we have not had for many years.

---

* See Lecture on Acclimation, by the author, delivered to and published by his class, when he occupied the chair of Theory and Practice of Medicine and Clinical Practice in the Medical College of Louisiana, in 1837.

APPENDIX.

I have been kindly supplied (and mainly through Mr. H. G. Heartt, Actuary of the Mutual Benefit Insurance Company of this city) with the subjoined tables and data for the calculations from the other life insurance offices in this city, and as they furnish a strong argument corroborating the statement I have made in the 'Report,' it affords me great pleasure to add them here. That position is briefly this: that this climate is not *lethale per se*, but has been made so by superadded or abused conditions — by circumstances extraneous to the physical condition; and this is demonstrated by the health of the neighborhood, the supervention of years of remarkable salubrity, and the great difference in the mortality of males and females in this city; that difference being sometimes 7, and sometimes as many as 13 to 1, in favor of females! arising mainly from difference in mode of life; being an eloquent testimony in favor of correct habits, in this respect, never to be overlooked. I now invite the attention of the reader to the singular fact — to show the influence of hygienic rules — that, whereas the mortality of the *whites* in this climate for the last two years (and select these because the mortality has been very large from cholera, etc., and they are of the same date as that embraced by the Insurance Companies) has been 9.83 per cent., or 1 in 10.36; and that of *negroes*, 3.44 per cent., or 1 in 29.66; while, by the materials furnished, this is entirely reversed, and the white mortality is actually only 0.77 of 1 per cent., while the negro is 1.72 per cent. (and most of the mortality has been produced by *cholera*). In these last cases, both may be considered as picked lives, although all the insured are of those ages most liable to death here, viz., middle life. The one really takes care of himself, for himself and family, while the other is reckless and indifferent to influences which the first so carefully avoids. So powerful do I consider the influence of proper habits in correcting the influence of climate or condition, that I place personal, paramount to general, hygiène:— the one is for the individual, (and is controlled by his sense of interest) what the other is for the community, who are ignorant of its importance, and here extremely negligent of it. A warm climate and a filthy city deteriorates health where their opposites would not, and although much personal care will, in a great measure, remove most of their influences, yet the mass fall victims to them. This opinion is not given at random -- I have the figures to sustain me; besides which, a professional acquaintance with the climate of thirty years, during all which time I have been collecting memoranda in relation to it, gives me full authority to speak boldly.

From the great difference, then, in the tables of general mortality and those of the special mortality, as furnished by the insurance companies, arise the profits of such companies. From this showing it is evident they must be greater here than in any part of the world! and I feel very sure that nowhere is there a greater difference in the prolonged enjoyments, as well as the hazards of life, between provident care and extreme recklessness.

E. H. BARTON.

MUTUAL BENEFIT LIFE AND FIRE INSURANCE COMPANY OF LOUISIANA.

A **TABULAR VIEW** of the Results of Life Insurance, as exemplified by the Experience of this Office, from its commencement to 1st April, 1851, a period of one year and nine months.

MEMORANDUM OF NUMBER INSURED, ETC.	PLACE OF BIRTH.	DISEASE.	AGE.	Whites.	Blacks.	TOTAL.
Of 716 Negroes insured in this Office, for a term of one year each, or less, 18 have died, making the proportion of deaths to the number insured, 2.513+ per cent. The ages of the insured ranging from 18@45 years.	Of the deceased, 1 was born in North Carolina; 5 " Kentucky; 2 " Virginia; 1 " Tennessee; 1 " Alabama; 1 " Louisiana; 1 " South Carolina; 6 " Unknown. —— 18	Cholera.........	14@19	..	3	
		Do.	20@24	..	2	
		Do.	25@29	..	1	
		Do.	30@34	..	1	
		Do.	35@39	..	0	
		Do.	40@44	..	1	8
		Phthisis pulmonalis.	20	..	1	
		Ditto	30	..	1	2
		Drowned.........	17	..	1	
		Do.	36	..	1	2
		Typhoid fever.....	23	..	1	1
		Ulceration of throat.	24	..	1	1
		Diarrhœa	30	..	1	1
		Endo-Carditis.....	32	..	1	1
		Gastro-Enteritis....	33	..	1	1
		Dropsy and paralysis,	45	..	1	1
		Deaths total of negroes........				18
Of 266 Whites insured, 48 for 1 year term, 1 deceased. 68 for 7 " 1 " 150 for Life .. 0 " —— 266 Making the proportion of deaths to the number insured, 0.75+ per cent. Ages of insured from 18 to 45 years.	New Orleans, La.	Retrocedent Gout, convalescent of severe Cholera,	34	1		1
	Kentucky	Cholera	33	1		1
		Deaths total of whites.........				2

MUTUAL BENEFIT LIFE INSURANCE COMPANY, NEWARK, NEW JERSEY.

A TABULAR VIEW of the Results of Life Insurance, as exemplified by the Experience of the Agency at New Orleans, from November, 1848, to June 1, 1851, a period of three years, under the supervision of

H. G. HEARTT, Agent.

PLACE OF BIRTH.	NUMBER.	AGES WHEN INSURED.		REMARKS.
		YEARS.	NUMBER.	
New York - - -	11	29	1	Of thirty-seven white persons insured during the existence of this Agency, covering risks to the amount of $198,000, not one death has occurred. It will be recollected that cholera prevailed during December, 1848, and a portion of 1849.
Pensylvania - - -	4	24	2	
Connecticut - -	4	26	1	
Massachusetts - -	3	30	1	
Kentucky - - -	3	31	3	
New Jersey - - -	2	32	1	
Rhode Island - -	1	33	4	
Tennessee - - -	1	34	4	
Mississippi - - -	1	35	3	
Alabama - - -	1	36	1	
England - - - -	2	37	4	
Ireland - - - -	1	38	6	
Germany - - - -	1	40	3	
West Indies - -	1	41	1	
Unknown - - - -	1	45	1	
		47	1	
TOTAL - -	37	....	37	

TABLE OF THE RATE OF MORTALITY AT CARLISLE,
Commonly known as the Carlisle Tables.

Age.	Number alive in each year	Deaths in that year.	Age.	Number alive in each year.	Deaths in that year	Age.	Number alive in each year.	Deaths in that year.
0	10000	1539	35	5362	55	70	2401	124
1	8461	682	36	5307	56	71	2277	134
2	7779	505	37	5251	57	72	2143	146
3	7274	276	38	5194	58	73	1997	156
4	6998	201	39	5136	61	74	1841	166
5	6797	121	40	5075	66	75	1675	160
6	6676	82	41	5009	69	76	1515	156
7	6594	58	42	4940	71	77	1359	146
8	6536	43	43	4869	71	78	1213	132
9	6493	33	44	4798	71	79	1081	128
10	6460	29	45	4727	70	80	953	116
11	6431	31	46	4657	69	81	837	112
12	6400	32	47	4588	67	82	725	102
13	6368	33	48	4521	63	83	623	94
14	6335	35	49	4458	61	84	529	84
15	6300	39	50	4397	59	85	445	78
16	6261	42	51	4338	62	86	367	71
17	6219	43	52	4276	65	87	296	64
18	6176	43	53	4211	68	88	232	51
19	6133	43	54	4143	70	89	181	39
20	6090	43	55	4073	73	90	142	37
21	6047	42	56	4000	76	91	105	30
22	6005	42	57	3924	82	92	75	21
23	5963	42	58	3842	93	93	54	14
24	5921	42	59	3749	106	94	40	10
25	5879	43	60	3643	122	95	30	7
26	5836	43	61	3521	126	96	23	5
27	5793	45	62	3395	127	97	18	4
28	5748	50	63	3268	125	98	14	3
29	5698	56	64	3143	125	99	11	2
30	5642	57	65	3018	124	100	9	2
31	5585	57	66	2894	123	101	7	2
32	5528	56	67	2771	123	102	5	2
33	5472	55	68	2648	123	103	3	2
34	5417	55	69	2525	124	104	1	1

TABLE, showing the probabilities of the Duration of Human Life at all Ages from 10 to 97, deduced from the experience of the Equitable Insurance Company, of London.

AGES.	LIVING.	DECRE-MENTS	AGES.	LIVING.	DECRE-MENTS	AGES.	LIVING.	DECRE-MENTS
10	5000	36	40	3922	43	70	1800	115
11	4964	36	41	3879	44	71	1685	115
12	4928	36	42	3835	44	72	1570	115
13	4892	36	43	3791	44	73	1455	115
14	4856	36	44	3747	45	74	1340	115
15	4820	36	45	3702	47	75	1225	114
16	4784	36	46	3655	47	76	1111	109
17	4748	36	47	3608	48	77	1002	105
18	4712	36	48	3560	49	78	897	101
19	4676	35	49	3511	50	79	796	96
20	4641	34	50	3461	52	80	700	93
21	4607	33	51	3409	55	81	607	90
22	4574	33	52	3354	58	82	517	85
23	4541	33	53	3296	62	83	432	83
24	4508	33	54	3234	64	84	349	73
25	4475	34	55	3170	66	85	276	61
26	4441	34	56	3104	70	86	215	50
27	4407	34	57	3034	75	87	165	42
28	4373	34	58	2959	79	88	123	34
29	4339	34	59	2880	84	89	89	22
30	4305	35	60	2796	88	90	67	18
31	4270	35	61	2708	90	91	49	14
32	4235	36	62	2618	91	92	35	11
33	4199	37	63	2527	93	93	24	8
34	4162	38	64	2434	95	94	16	7
35	4124	38	65	2339	100	95	9	5
36	4086	39	66	2239	105	96	4	3
37	4047	40	67	2134	108	97	1	1
38	4007	42	68	2026	111		244092	5000
39	3965	43	69	1915	115			

TABLE OF THE NEW RATE OF MORTALITY IN ENGLAND:

Exhibiting the LAW OF MORTALITY AMONGST ASSURED LIVES, according to the combined Town and Country Experience of Life Offices, deduced from 62,537 Assurances under the superintendence of a Committee of eminent Actuaries in London.

Completed Age.	Number Surviving at each Age.	Deaths in each Year.	Logarithm of Number surviving at each Age.	Completed Age.	Number Surviving at each Age.	Deaths in each Year.	Logarithm of Number surviving at each Age.
10	100000	676	5.0000000	55	63469	1375	4.8025617
11	99324	674	4.9970542	56	62094	1436	4.7930496
12	98650	672	4.9940971	57	60658	1497	4.7828881
13	97978	671	4.9911286	58	59161	1561	4.7720355
14	97307	671	4.9881441	59	57600	1627	4.7604225
15	96636	671	4.9851389	60	55973	1698	4.7479786
16	95965	672	4.9821129	61	54275	1770	4.7345998
17	95293	673	4.9790610	62	52505	1814	4.7202007
18	94620	675	4.9759829	63	50661	1917	4.7046738
19	93945	677	4.9728737	64	48744	1990	4.6879212
20	93268	680	4.9697327	65	46754	2061	4.6698188
21	92588	683	4.9665547	66	44693	2128	4.6502395
22	91905	686	4.9633391	67	42565	2191	4.6290526
23	91219	690	4.9600853	68	40374	2246	4.6061018
24	90529	694	4.9567877	69	38128	2291	4.5812440
25	89835	698	4.9534456	70	35837	2327	4.5543316
26	89137	703	4.9500580	71	33510	2351	4.5251744
27	88434	708	4.9466193	72	31159	2362	4.4935835
28	87726	714	4.9431283	73	28797	2358	4.4593472
29	87012	720	4.9395792	74	26439	2339	4.4222450
30	86292	727	4.9359705	75	24100	2303	4.3820170
31	85565	734	4.9322962	76	21797	2249	4.3383967
32	84831	742	4.9285546	77	19548	2179	4.2911023
33	84089	750	4.9247392	78	17369	2092	4.2397748
34	83339	758	4.9208483	79	15277	1987	4.1840311
35	82581	767	4.9168801	80	13290	1866	4.1235250
36	81814	776	4.9128276	81	11424	1730	4.0578182
37	81038	785	4.9086887	82	9694	1582	3.9865030
38	80253	795	4.9044613	83	8112	1427	3.9091279
39	79458	805	4.9001376	84	6685	1268	3.8251014
40	78653	815	4.8957153	85	5417	1111	3.7337588
41	77838	826	4.8911917	86	4306	958	3.6340740
42	77012	839	4.8865584	87	3348	811	3.5247854
43	76173	857	4.8818011	88	2537	673	3.4043205
44	75316	881	4.8768872	89	1864	545	3.2404459
45	74435	909	4.8717772	90	1319	427	3.1202448
46	73526	944	4.8664409	91	892	322	2.9503649
47	72582	981	4.8608289	92	570	231	2.7558749
48	71601	1021	4.8549191	93	339	155	2.5301997
49	70580	1063	4.8486817	94	184	95	2.2648178
50	69517	1108	4.8420910	95	89	52	1.9493900
51	68409	1156	4.8351132	96	37	24	1.5682017
52	67253	1207	4.8277117	97	13	9	1.1139434
53	66046	1261	4.8198465	98	4	3	0.6020600
54	64785	1316	4.8114745	99	1	1	0.0000000

TABLE, showing the DISORDERS (as certified to the Court of Directors) of which persons assured by the Equitable Society have died during thirty-two years, from the 1st of January, 1801, to the 31st December, 1832.

DISEASES.	10 TO 20	20 TO 30	30 TO 40	40 TO 50	50 TO 60	60 TO 70	70 TO 80	80 ETC	Total
Accidents	..	7	..	11	9	4	5	4	40
Angina pectoris	..	..	8	16	45	47	26	3	145
Aneurism	..	..	1	2	..	..	1	..	4
Apoplexy	1	4	25	56	129	169	86	16	486
Asthma	..	..	..	2	20	26	22	4	74
Atrophy	..	..	4	7	11	15	6	..	43
Cancer	..	..	2	5	14	15	4	3	43
Child-birth	..	..	2	2	..	..	..	..	4
Cholera morbus	..	..	2	5	5	9	5	1	27
Consumption	4	23	63	83	81	66	18	1	339
Convulsion fits	..	..	..	4	1	3	..	..	8
Decay (natural, and old age)	..	..	..	..	10	128	241	187	566
Diabetes	..	..	..	3	2	1	1	1	8
Disorders not properly defined	..	..	9	11	20	27	12	..	79
Dropsy	1	..	10	39	67	83	50	7	257
Dropsy on the chest	..	1	3	23	52	59	42	3	183
Dysentery	..	..	1	3	5	11	11	3	34
Disease of the stomach and digestive organs	..	2	9	12	28	31	22	2	106
Diseased liver	..	2	8	37	54	49	23	2	175
Disease of the bladder and urinary passages	..	..	2	9	25	44	41	6	128
Epilepsy	..	1	2	8	2	2	4	..	19
Erysipelas	..	1	2	7	6	7	3	..	26
Fevers, general	..	5	30	55	61	70	34	7	262
" bilious	..	1	5	10	10	8	2	1	37
" nervous	..	3	3	13	9	9	5	..	42
" inflammatory	..	3	2	6	10	5	6	..	32
" putrid	..	2	7	4	7	7	1	..	28
Gout	..	..	2	6	8	14	7	1	38
Inflammation of the bowels	2	2	14	20	26	44	16	2	126
" of the lungs	..	2	12	12	41	56	45	17	185
" of the brain	1	4	15	16	13	12	2	1	64
Inflammation of the chest and peripneumony	1	1	1	8	11	21	12	4	59
Mortification	..	..	..	2	12	14	12	6	46
Murdered	..	..	..	1	1	..	1	..	3
Palsy	..	1	5	15	47	84	74	9	235
Pleurisy	..	..	..	1	1	2	..	..	4
Quincy	..	..	..	1	1	1	..	..	3
Rupture of a blood vessel	1	..	12	19	19	22	6	..	82
Slain in War	1	1	1	1	..	..	..	..	4
Small-pox	..	..	..	..	..	..	..	1	1
Stone	..	..	..	..	1	2	7	2	12
Suicide	..	1	2	6	15	5	..	..	29
Water on the brain	..	..	1	3	4	1	..	..	9
	12	67	266	544	883	1173	856	294	4095

TABLE OF COMPARATIVE EXPECTATIONS OF LIFE IN ENGLAND.

Showing the Expectation or Average duration of Life, deduced from Eight Original Tables prepared under the Superintendence of a committee of eminent Actuaries, and compared with the Carlisle, Equitable and Northampton Tables.

COMPLETED AGE.	MALE LIVES—Town, Country and Irish Experience.	FEMALE LIVES—Town, Country and Irish Experience.	Town Experience.	Country Experience.	Irish Experience.	Combined Town Experience.	General Experience.	Adjusted Experience.	CARLISLE Experience.	EQUITABLE Experience.	NORTHAMPTON Experience.	COMPLETED AGE.
20	39.84	35.86	41.22	40.33	34.95	41.55	40.97	41.49	41.46	41.06	33.43	20
21	39.29	36.01	40.68	40.29	34.48	40.96	40.45	40.79	40.75	40.33	32.90	21
22	38.70	36.20	40.47	39.89	33.48	40.38	39.92	40.09	40.04	39.60	32.39	22
23	37.98	35.41	39.87	38.98	32.78	39.65	39.18	39.39	39.31	38.88	31.88	23
24	37.41	34.81	39.23	38.37	32.64	38.98	38.54	38.68	38.59	38.16	31.36	24
25	36.63	34.41	38.56	37.55	31.94	38.26	37.84	37.98	37.86	37.44	30.85	25
26	35.88	33.79	37.82	36.88	31.05	37.54	37.13	37.27	37.14	36.73	30.33	26
27	35.23	33.14	37.10	36.12	30.99	36.84	36.42	36.56	36.41	36.02	29.82	27
28	34.63	33.07	36.45	35.54	30.76	36.12	35.76	35.86	35.69	35.33	29.30	28
29	33.96	32.61	35.67	34.91	30.56	35.38	35.06	35.15	35.00	34.65	28.79	29
30	33.17	31.73	34.84	34.20	29.71	34.54	34.25	34.43	34.34	33.38	28.27	30
31	32.44	31.04	34.07	33.51	29.08	33.78	33.50	33.72	33.68	33.40	27.76	31
32	31.73	30.51	33.34	32.86	28.36	33.01	32.75	33.01	33.03	32.64	27.24	32
33	30.92	29.86	32.53	32.05	27.63	32.22	31.98	32.20	32.36	31.98	26.72	33
34	30.21	29.60	31.87	31.41	26.85	31.51	31.27	31.58	31.68	31.32	26.20	34
35	29.52	29.07	31.12	30.78	26.30	30.77	30.55	30.87	31.00	30.66	25.68	35
36	28.87	28.88	30.44	30.20	25.77	30.08	29.90	30.15	30.32	30.01	25.16	36
37	28.15	28.30	29.69	29.45	25.26	29.37	29.20	29.44	29.64	29.35	24.64	37
38	27.49	27.62	29.00	28.81	24.61	28.65	28.51	28.72	28.96	28.70	24.12	38
39	26.81	27.00	28.34	28.16	23.93	27.92	27.79	28.00	28.28	28.05	23.60	39
40	26.06	26.36	27.53	27.38	23.36	27.20	27.07	27.28	27.61	27.40	23.08	40
41	25.42	25.84	26.85	26.73	22.86	26.51	26.41	26.56	26.97	26.74	22.56	41
42	24.70	25.34	26.19	26.01	22.14	25.79	25.68	25.84	26.34	26.07	22.04	42
43	24.00	24.57	25.47	25.22	21.56	25.07	24.93	25.12	25.71	25.40	21.54	43
44	23.34	23.94	24.77	24.59	21.00	24.32	24.26	24.40	25.09	24.75	21.03	44
45	22.63	23.21	24.08	23.83	20.30	23.61	23.55	23.69	24.46	24.10	20.52	45
46	21.98	22.60	23.42	23.13	19.76	22.90	22.85	22.97	23.82	23.44	20.02	46
47	21.24	21.97	22.70	22.34	19.12	22.15	22.12	22.27	23.17	22.78	19.51	47
48	20.62	21.16	22.01	21.67	18.59	21.44	21.41	21.56	22.50	22.12	19.00	48
49	20.08	20.69	21.34	21.13	18.27	20.77	20.79	20.87	21.81	21.47	18.49	49

TABLE OF COMPARATIVE EXPECTATIONS OF LIFE IN ENGLAND — (Continued.)

COMPLETED AGE.	MALE LIVES — Town, Country and Irish Experience.	FEMALE LIVES — Town, Country and Irish Experience.	Town Experience.	Country Experience.	Irish Experience.	Combined Town Experience.	General Experience.	Adjusted Experience.	CARLISLE Experience.	EQUITABLE Experience.	NORTHAMPTON Experience.	COMPLETED AGE.
50	19.41	20.05	20.58	20.48	17.76	20.07	20.11	20.18	21.11	20.83	17.99	50
51	18.73	19.46	19.89	19.73	17.20	19.41	19.46	19.50	20.39	20.20	17.50	51
52	18.05	18.80	19.17	19.03	16.62	18.75	18.79	18.82	19.68	19.59	17.02	52
53	17.40	18.31	18.52	18.30	16.11	18.11	18.16	18.16	18.97	19.00	16.54	53
54	16.77	17.58	17.95	17.55	15.51	17.46	17.50	17.50	18.28	18.43	16.06	54
55	16.21	16.78	17.25	16.96	15.04	16.76	16.83	16.86	17.58	17.85	15.58	55
56	15.66	16.07	16.74	16.40	14.41	16.17	16.23	16.22	16.89	17.28	15.10	56
57	15.09	15.39	16.08	15.87	13.85	15.56	15.62	15.59	16.21	16.71	14.63	57
58	14.45	14.79	15.35	15.24	13.34	14.90	14.98	14.97	15.55	16.15	14.15	58
59	13.99	14.28	14.86	14.60	13.04	14.25	14.38	14.47	14.92	15.60	13.68	59
60	13.47	13.78	14.23	14.03	12.67	13.68	13.81	13.77	14.34	15.06	13.21	60
61	12.99	13.10	13.58	13.50	12.29	13.08	13.24	13.18	13.82	14.51	12.75	61
62	12.46	12.41	13.01	12.87	11.81	12.52	12.68	12.61	13.31	13.96	12.28	62
63	11.90	11.87	12.26	12.26	11.45	11.91	12.09	12.05	12.81	13.42	11.81	63
64	11.27	11.09	11.62	11.75	10.67	11.32	11.50	11.51	12.30	12.88	11.35	64
65	10.87	10.60	11.18	11.44	10.19	10.86	11.03	10.97	11.79	12.35	10.88	65
66	10.38	10.00	10.69	10.82	9.74	10.37	10.51	10.46	11.27	11.83	10.42	66
67	9.93	9.56	10.11	10.26	9.44	9.87	10.03	9.96	10.75	11.32	9.96	67
68	9.33	8.85	9.57	9.72	8.73	9.31	9.46	9.47	10.23	10.82	9.50	68
69	8.81	8.38	9.29	8.94	8.27	8.88	8.99	9.00	9.70	10.32	9.05	69
70	8.34	7.93	8.61	8.48	7.92	8.44	8.50	8.54	9.18	9.84	8.60	70
71	7.88	7.31	8.33	7.92	7.37	8.10	8.13	8.10	8.65	9.36	8.17	71
72	7.43	6.63	7.65	7.37	6.98	7.69	7.72	7.67	8.16	8.88	7.74	72
73	6.97	6.19	7.08	6.76	6.70	7.22	7.26	7.26	7.72	8.42	7.33	73
74	6.57	5.72	6.53	6.31	6.37	6.79	6.84	6.86	7.33	7.97	6.92	74
75	6.03	5.37	6.29	5.55	5.97	6.45	6.46	6.48	7.01	7.52	6.54	75
76	5.63	5.45	6.34	5.45	5.34	6.10	6.08	6.11	6.69	7.08	6.18	76
77	5.48	4.78	5.52	4.90	5.59	5.74	5.77	5.76	6.40	6.64	5.83	77
78	5.16	4.56	5.19	4.69	5.23	5.39	5.37	5.42	6.12	6.20	5.48	78
79	4.99	4.80	5.32	4.91	4.80	5.05	5.07	5.09	5.80	5.78	5.11	79
80	4.75	4.75	4.75	4.75	4.75	4.75	4.75	4.78	5.51	5.38	4.75	80

SEVENTH CENSUS.
POPULATION OF THE UNITED STATES—APPORTIONMENT OF REPRESENTATIVES.

STATES.	WHITE POPULATION.	FREE COLORED POPULATION.	TOTAL FREE.	SLAVES.	FEDERAL REPRESENTATIVE POPULATION.	NUMBER OF REP'S.	FRACTIONS.
Alabama	426,515	2,250	428,765	342,894	634,501	6	*72,289
Arkansas	126,071	587	162,658	46,983	190,848	2	3,444
California	200,000	—	200,000	—	200,000	2	12,596
Connecticut	363,189	7,415	370,604	—	370,604	3	*89,498
Delaware	71,282	17,957	89,239	2,289	906,612	—	*90,612
Florida	47,120	926	48,046	39,341	71,650	—	*71,650
Georgia	513,083	2,586	515,669	362,966	733,448	7	*77,534
Indiana	983,634	5,100	988,734	—	988,734	10	*51,714
Illinois	853,059	5,239	858,298	—	858,298	9	20,980
Iowa	191,830	292	192,122	—	192,122	2	4,718
Kentucky	770,061	9,667	779,728	221,768	912,788	9	*75,470
Louisiana	254,271	15,685	269,955	230,807	408,440	4	33,632
Maine	581,920	1,312	583,232	—	583,232	6	21,020
Massachusetts	985,498	8,773	994,271	—	984,271	10	*57,251
Maryland	418,763	73,943	492,706	89,800	546,586	5	*78,076
Mississippi	291,536	898	292,434	300,419	472,685	4	4,175
Michigan	393,156	2,517	395,703	—	395,703	5	20,895
Missouri	592,176	2,667	594,843	89,289	648,416	6	*86,204
New Hampshire	317,354	477	317,831	—	317,831	3	36,725
New York	3,042,574	47,448	3,090,022	—	2,090,022	32	*91,558
New Jersey	466,283	22,269	488,552	119	488,623	5	20,113
North Carolina	552,477	27,271	†580,458	288,412	735,505	8	3,889
Ohio	1,951,101	25,930	1,977,031	—	1,977,031	21	9,289
Pennsylvania	2,258,480	53,201	2,311,681	—	2,311,681	24	*62,533
Rhode Island	144,012	3,543	147,555	—	147,555	1	*53,853
South Carolina	274,775	8,769	283,544	384,925	514,499	5	45,989
Tennessee	767,319	6,280	773,599	249,519	923,310	9	*89,992
Texas	133,131	926	134,057	53,346	166,064	1	*72,362
Vermont	312,756	710	313,466	—	313,466	3	32,360
Virginia	894,149	53,906	948,055	473,026	1,231,870	13	13,744
Wisconsin	303,600	626	304,226	—	304,226	3	23,120
	19,517,885	409,200	19,927,085	2,173,902			
Dist. of Columbia	38,027	9,973	48,000	3,687			
TERRITORIES.							
Minnesota	6,192	—	6,192				
New Mexico	61,632	—	61,632				
Oregon	20,000	—	20,000				
Utah	25,000	—	25,000				
	19,668,736	419,173	20,087,909	3,175,589	21,832,621	218	
Representatives allowed for fractional numbers, as marked						15	
Whole number of representatives under the next apportionment						233	

* These States have a representative added to the number of apportionment.
† Including 710 civilized Indians.

RECAPITULATION.

	TOTAL FREE POPULATION.	SLAVES.	REPRESENTATIVE POPULATION.
Free States	13,533,326	119	13,533,399
Slave States	6,393,757	3,175,783	8,299,226
Districts and Territories	160,824	3,687	
	20,087,909	3,179,589	21,832,625
Total free population			20,087,909
Slaves			3,179,589
			23,267,498
Ratio of representation			93,702

CHART No. 1.

CLIMATE OF LOUISIANA,

As exhibited in **New Orleans,** Latitude 30° North: Mean Annual Temperature in 1807–'10, = 70° 29′, and in 1833–'50, = 67° 52′. . . . . ie Annual Averages of Rain in 1833–'50 = 52.330 inches — 13 years
Do. in **West Feliciana,** " 30° 38′ Do. do. in 1820–'33, = 65° 83′. . . . . Do. do. in 1820–'33 = 61.344 " — 13 "
Do. in **Rapides,** " 31° 08′ Do. do. in 1833–'39, = 65° 50′, and in 1848–'50, = 68° 10′. or of both = 66° 80′. Do. do. in 1848–'50 = 67.400 " — 3 "
Do. in **Plaquemine,** " 29° 50′ Do. do. in 1845–'50 = 67.080 " — 6 "

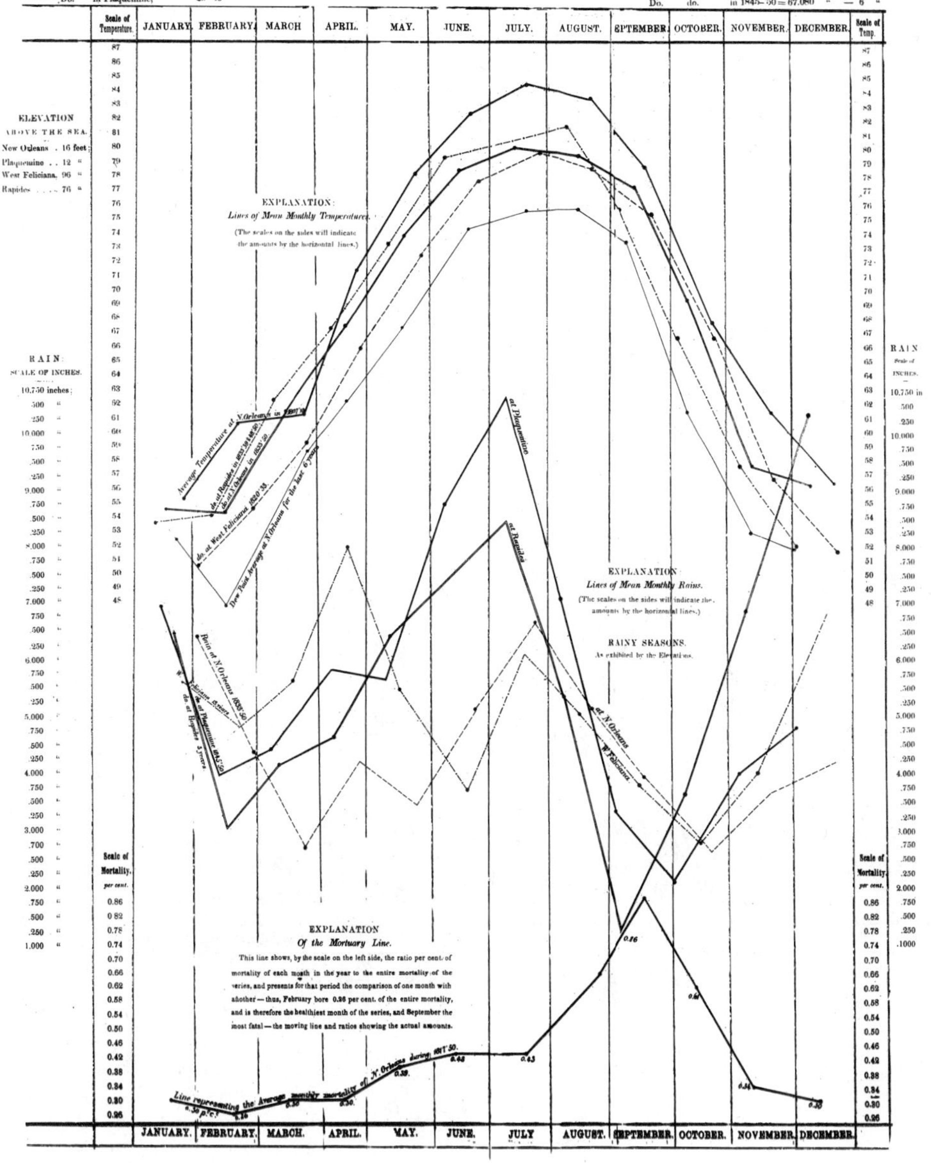

CHART No. II.

CLIMATE OF NEW ORLEANS AND LAFAYETTE.

EFFECT ON RACES AND SEX, as exhibited in the Mortality of Whites — Male and Female — and the Colored Population, with the Total Mortality for 1850.

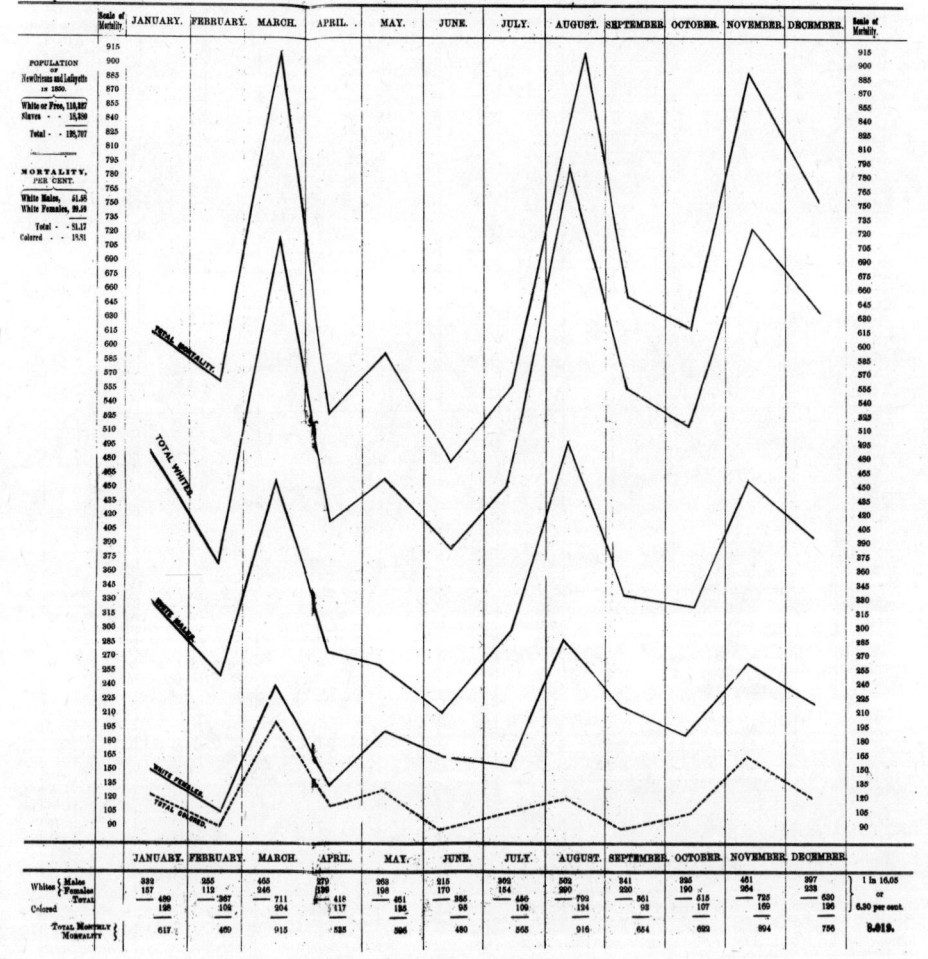

CHART No. III.

INFLUENCE OF CLIMATE ON RACES,

As exhibited in the Mortality of the Whites and Colored in New Orleans in 1849 — of the same ages.

TABLE:

Explanation: — The horizontal lines will show on each side the actual monthly mortality of each color of the same age by the scale.

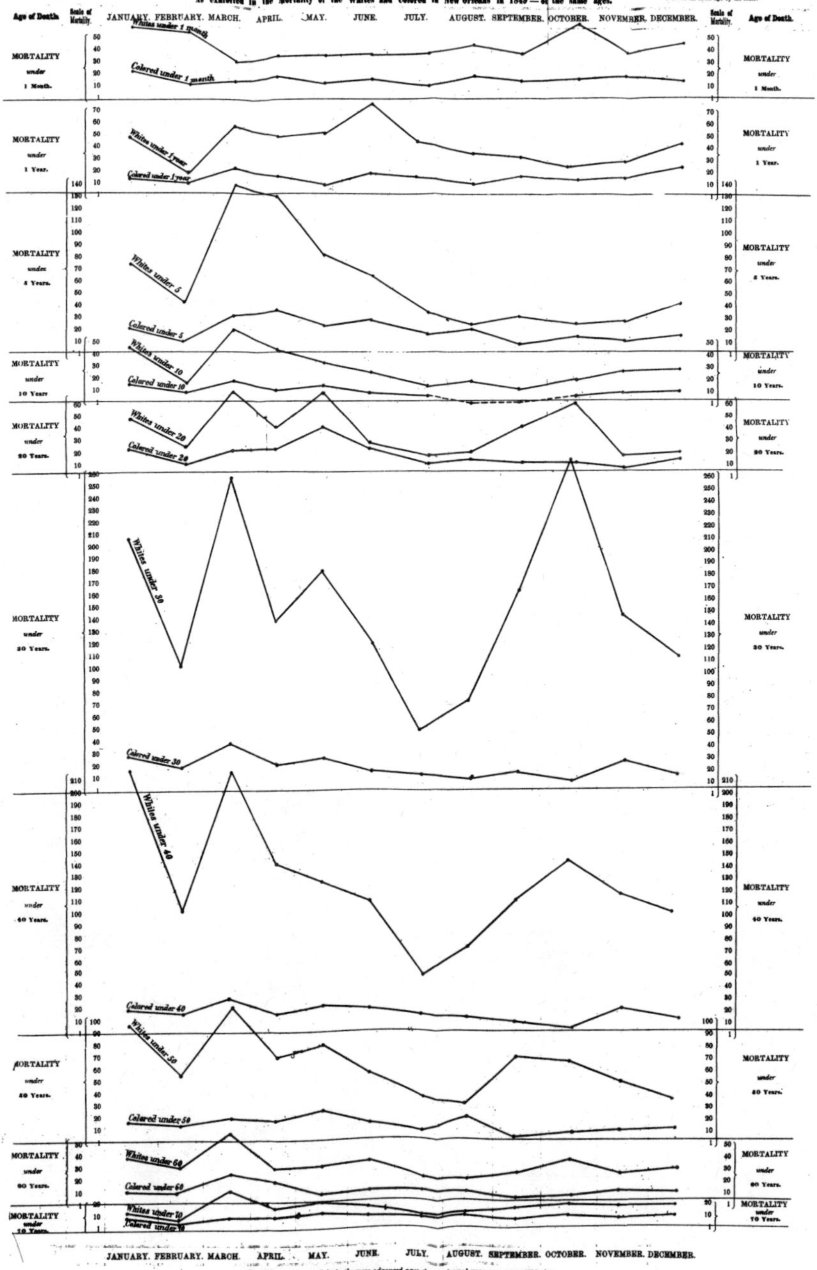

The differences are so slight in *the more advanced ages*, that it is deemed unnecessary to exhibit them.

Probable population in 1849: { Whites, 71,028, Colored, 47,352, } 118,380. Ratios of mortality: { Whites, 1 in 8.88, or 11.24; Colored, 1 in 25.14, or 3.97.

ORGANIZATION, ACTIVITIES, AND RESULTS UP TO DECEMBER 31, 1910

[Wickliffe Rose]

THE ROCKEFELLER SANITARY COMMISSION

FOR THE

ERADICATION OF HOOKWORM DISEASE

ORGANIZATION, ACTIVITIES, AND RESULTS

UP TO DECEMBER 31, 1910

OFFICES OF THE COMMISSION
WASHINGTON, D. C.
1910

THE ROCKEFELLER SANITARY COMMISSION

F. T. GATES
Chairman

L. G. MYERS
Treasurer

WILLIAM H. WELCH	J. Y. JOYNER
SIMON FLEXNER	WALTER H. PAGE
E. A. ALDERMAN	H. B. FRISSELL
D. F. HOUSTON	J. D. ROCKEFELLER, JR.
P. P. CLAXTON	STARR J. MURPHY
WICKLIFFE ROSE	C. W. STILES
Administrative Secretary	*Scientific Secretary*
811 Union Trust Building	24th and E streets N. W.
Washington, D. C.	Washington, D. C.

ORGANIZATION, ACTIVITIES, AND RESULTS UP TO DECEMBER 31, 1910.

The Rockefeller Sanitary Commission for the eradication of hookworm disease was organized October 26, 1909. By informal action of the Executive Committee an administrative secretary was appointed in December, 1909. On January 8, 1910, offices were opened in the Union Trust Building, in Washington, D. C., and the more definite organization of the work was begun.

I. **The work to be done.**—The Commission had been created for the purpose of eradicating hookworm disease. To do this involved undertaking three definite tasks: To determine the geographic distribution of the infection and to make a reliable estimate of the degree of infection for each infected area; to cure the present sufferers; and, finally, to remove the source of infection by putting a stop to soil pollution.

II. **Organizing the agency to do this work.**—The State was adopted as the unit of organization and of work. It was regarded as fundamental in the interest both of economy and of efficiency that the work be done as far as possible through existing agencies. Each State has its own system of public health, its own system of organized medicine, its own organized public press, its own system of public schools—these four fundamentals and a host of minor agencies which can be used to advantage in educating the people. These are established institutions rooted in the life and traditions of the people; to enlist these agencies in the accomplishment of the task is to insure the permanency of the work from the beginning.

The eradication of this disease, moreover, is a work which no outside agency working independently could do for a people if it would, and one which no outside agency should do if it could. The economic prosperity of the State, the lives and health of its people, and the education of its children are involved; if the infection is to be stamped out, the States in which it exists must assume the responsibility. An outside agency can be helpful only in so far as it aids the States in organizing and bringing into activity their own forces.

In this spirit the Commission responded to invitations from State boards of health to coöperate in organizing the work in those States in which widespread infection had been demonstrated. The nucleus of this organization comprises:

1. **A State Director of Sanitation.**—This man is appointed by the joint action of the State public health authorities and the Rockefeller Sanitary Commission. He is a State official, an officer of the State department of health, and is clothed with the powers and responsibilities belonging to such position. He is the organizing and directing head of the whole work for the eradication of hookworm disease in his State, and is responsible for the efficiency of the service. His work is done under the general supervision of the State department of health; he reports quarterly to the State department and through this department to the Commission. These reports are manifolded, bound together, and sent to each man in the service. The admin-

istrative secretary of the Commission is kept in constant touch with the details of the work by correspondence and personal observation.

On this basis a State director of sanitation* has been appointed and the work inaugurated in the following States:

State.	State Director of Sanitation.	Work inaugurated.
Virginia	A. W. Freeman	February 7, 1910
North Carolina	John A. Ferrell	March 12, 1910
Georgia	A. G. Fort	April 20, 1910
South Carolina	J. La Bruce Ward	May 1, 1910
Tennessee	Olin West	May 10, 1910
Arkansas	Morgan Smith	May 10, 1910
Mississippi	W. S. Leathers	June 1, 1910
Alabama	W. W. Dinsmore	October 1, 1910
Louisiana	Sidney D. Porter	November 1, 1910

2. **A field force of sanitary inspectors.**—Under the direct supervision of each State director of sanitation is a force of sanitary inspectors. These inspectors are nominated by the State director of sanitation and confirmed by the joint action of the State department of health and the Sanitary Commission. These inspectors constitute an ambulant service and devote their whole time to work in the field. They are the long arms with which the State director reaches out over the State to determine the geographic distribution and degree of infection; to determine the sanitary conditions responsible for the presence and spread of the disease; to enlist the coöperation of the physicians in curing the sufferers; to provide for the treatment of the indigent; to inspect the schools; to instruct the teachers, enlist the

---

* The official title varies in some States to conform to State usage.

press, and, by lectures, demonstrations, and personal conference, teach the people the importance of getting all infected persons cured, and how to prevent the spread of the disease by putting a stop to soil pollution.

The sanitary inspectors report daily to the State director of sanitation. For this, and for other reports made at longer intervals, forms are supplied. Each inspector is supplied with microscope, medicine, literature, lantern, and slides. The sanitary inspectors by States are: VIRGINIA, A. C. Fisher, W. A. Brumfield, R. C. Carnal, W. A. Plecker; NORTH CAROLINA, B. W. Page, C. F. Strosnider, C. L. Pridgen; SOUTH CAROLINA, F. A. Bell, Milton Weinberg; GEORGIA, C. E. Pattillo, C. H. Dobbs, P. H. Fitzgerald, S. H. Jacobs, W. C. Thompson, T. F. Abercrombie; ALABAMA, H. G. Perry, John F. Orr, W. W. Perdue; MISSISSIPPI, W. H. Rowan, C. R. Stingily, R. N. Whitfield, J. C. Cully, Robert Rowland; TENNESSEE, T. B. Yancey, Jr., W. M. Breeding, W. J. Breeding, J. M. Lee; ARKANSAS, C. C. Price, J. B. Crawford; LOUISIANA, no appointments made as yet.

3. **Laboratory staff.**—A definite diagnosis of hookworm disease requires a microscopic examination of the patient's stool. One person can make from twenty to thirty-five such examinations a day. Each State has offered to make these examinations without charge. This requires a State laboratory with microscopes and men enough to examine the specimens that are sent in.

At the beginning of the work each State, except Arkansas, Mississippi, and Tennessee, was maintaining a public-health laboratory with staff and equipment more or less adequate. But, as the influence of the work extends, as larger numbers of physicians and of people become interested, the work of the State laboratory grows, and calls for a corresponding increase in the staff.

The North Carolina State laboratory, which ten months ago needed no special staff for this service, now has five men devoting their whole time to examining specimens for hookworm disease, and has applied for two additional men to keep up with the work. Virginia has in this service one laboratory man; Mississippi, one; Alabama, two; Georgia, two; Louisiana, one, and South Carolina, one.

This definite organization devoted exclusively to this service is relied upon to enlist in the accomplishment of its task the physicians, the press, the schools, and all forces in the State which may be used as agencies in educating the people.

III. **The organization at work.**—The work in each State has been directed toward the accomplishment of three definite tasks:

1. **Determining the geographic distribution of the infection and estimating the degree of infection for each infected area.**—The survey to determine the infection is made by counties. The State director of sanitation first makes a preliminary survey to locate the infection and to determine roughly whether it is "heavy" or "light." This is followed later, in connection with the other features of the work, with a survey in detail, which estimates what percentage of the total population is infected. The plans followed in making these surveys vary in details; the essentials are these:

(1) **Personal inspection.**—The State Director, on taking up his duties, goes into the field and makes a tour of personal inspection through those counties in which heaviest infection is suspected. He consults physicians, sees a few of their patients, inspects the children in schools, observes the people along the roads, at railroad stations, in country churches, and in the market places of country towns. His hurried clinical diagnosis he checks up by occasional microscopic examinations.

When in this way he has located a large area showing heavy infection, he creates a sanitary district comprising four or five counties, appoints a sanitary inspector to take up the work in detail in this district, and continues his preliminary survey in new territory. In the end the State director and his inspectors, who are frequently assigned temporarily to this duty, will have made a personal preliminary survey of every county in the State.

(2) **Reports from local physicians.**—The State director sends a personal letter to the physicians of the State, asking each one to report the cases of hookworm disease which he has diagnosed and treated. This letter is persistently followed up. As the physicians learn to recognize and treat the disease, these reports grow in number and in value. Dr. Ferrell, of North Carolina, has received reports of about 8,000 cases treated by physicians in 94 out of the 98 counties in the State.

(3) **Laboratory examinations.**—By systematic planning the laboratory records are made to indicate both distribution and **degree** of infection. The work done in two States makes this clear:

a. All miscellaneous specimens examined are recorded on the State map, thus showing distribution of infection.

b. Three hundred college students were examined as a body without reference to clinical symptoms; the records were mapped by counties. The results showed infection in 54 of the 98 counties in the State, and showed an infection of 42 per cent for this body of men.

c. The three regiments of the State militia and the coast artillery were examined; specimens were collected from all the men; records were made by counties and results mapped. The records show 1,105 men examined. Percentage of infection for First Regiment, 36.8; Second Regiment, 58; Third Regiment, 32; Naval Reserves, 30. Infection located in 34 counties, and percentage for the company in each county given.

d. Examinations of specimens from all the children in an orphanage gave as result: number of children examined, 96; age, 6 to 18 years; percentage of infection, 54; infection located in 21 counties. Other orphanages and State institutions were examined in like manner.

e. One public school was selected at random in each district in the county and specimens secured from all the children in each school selected. Records were made by schools. The results show an average infection of 82.6 per cent for all schools examined. This result, being based on an examination of children in school, is taken as conservative estimate of the average infection for all school children in the county.

The possibilities of the laboratory as a means of determining distribution and degree of infection are limited only by our laboratory facilities and our ingenuity in planning and conducting investigations.

(4) **Survey in detail by the sanitary inspectors.**—The sanitary inspector is an indispensable factor in this survey at every point. He aids the State director in making preliminary surveys of new territory; he enlists the coöperation of physicians and gets them to report conditions and cases treated in their practice; he secures specimens for systematic examinations being conducted at the laboratory; and, finally, he completes the work by a survey in detail of the sanitary district to which he is assigned. This detailed work he does not do as a thing by itself and at one time; he does it in connection with his other duties, and prolongs it with many interruptions over a long period of time. Dr. Fisher, the first sanitary inspector appointed, says he thinks he has located every focus of infection in the county in which he began his work last spring, and his knowledge of conditions in the other counties is growing toward complete mastery of his district.

To cover the State in this way will require years; but it will be done.

(5) **Summary of results showing:**

a. *Infection in nine States.*—Maps 1 to 9 show the results of the survey as made up to December 31, 1910. Infection has been demonstrated in every county marked infected. Heavy infection has been demonstrated in every county in which heavy infection is shown on the map. Where the infection is marked as light, a careful survey has demonstrated a light infection; where only the presence of infection is indicated, the degree of infection has not been determined.

b. Infection in other States.—In addition to the nine States in which the work has been organized, infection has been demonstrated in Florida, Kentucky, Texas, Oklahoma, California, and Nevada. It is reported as heavy and producing great economic loss in the mines of California.

c. Infection in foreign countries.—The Commission is getting information on conditions in foreign countries. In addition to learning what countries are infected, information is being sought on: 1, the geographic distribution of the infection within the country; 2, an approximate estimate of the degree of infection; 3, whether the infection is surface or mine infection; 4, what is being done by private or public agencies to eradicate or relieve it. The investigation is just getting well under way. Maps 10 to 15 show the countries in which hookworm infection has been demonstrated.

2. **Getting the sufferers cured.**—In getting the sufferers cured the State director and his staff follow three lines of effort: Enlisting the physicians in the accomplishment of the task; getting the people to seek examination and treatment, if needed, for themselves and their neighbors; providing for the treatment of the indigent.

(1) **Enlisting the physicians in the work.**—The State board of health in each State depends upon the physicians of the State to treat all cases of hookworm disease as it depends upon them to treat other diseases. This is a part of their practice; the State board would not take it from them. The task is enormous; it will require years for its accomplishment. It will be done only by the doctors working intelligently, patiently, persistently, each in his own territory.

There are in the nine States 19,981 physicians. These men are distributed over 415,950 square miles of territory. This disease is new to the profession; when the work began a year ago comparatively few physicians in these States were treating it. One of the definite tasks of the State organizations is to enlist this army of 20,000 men as a permanent working force. This is being done—

a. By bulletins.—Each State board of health publishes and distributes to all the physicians in its State special bulletins and folders on diagnosis and treatment of hookworm disease; it publishes special articles on the subject in its regular bulletin, which reaches all physicians in the State.

b. By letters.—The State director of sanitation makes personal appeal by letter to all the physicians of his State. These vary indefinitely in character, but the end is one—to get the physicians enlisted in the work.

c. By lectures.—The State director and his staff give lectures and demonstrations at the medical colleges, at the meetings of State, district, and county medical societies. Often an entire session at these meetings is given to a symposium on hookworm disease with a clinic as central feature.

d. By personal visits.—The sanitary inspector, on going into a new county, visits personally all the physicians; goes with them in their practice; gives demonstrations in diagnosis and treatment when desired; establishes personal relationships, and makes plans for permanent coöperation in the work.

(2) **Getting the people to seek examination and treatment.**—In Porto Rico it is not uncommon to see from one to two hundred people assembled at an anemia station wait-

ing each his turn to be examined and treated for hookworm disease, or "anemia," as they call it on the island. Many of these people, for whom exertion of any kind is difficult, have walked for miles over rugged mountain trails to see the doctor. They are eager to be treated, because for generations they have known anemia as a dread disease; it has been the scourge of the island. The infection is severe; the people are sick, they know they are sick, and have learned that they can be cured.

In the States the infection is less severe; it is scattered over larger areas; its effects have not been so perceptible to the people. They have taken their anemia, their lack of vitality, their feeling "puny" and "out of sorts," as a matter of course. Those that have been severely sick have been treated for malaria, tuberculosis, dropsy, kidney trouble, chronic indigestion, etc.; but hookworm disease, as a disease, has not been known to the people or to the profession. The announcement that hookworm is prevalent in the States was not taken seriously. Many people resented the suggestion of their being infected and refused to be examined and treated, even when they knew they were ill and when every indication pointed to hookworm disease. But, as the people get possession of the fact that hookworm infection is a reality; that all people are subject to it; that its consequences are serious; they come to look upon it as they have been accustomed to look upon tuberculosis, typhoid fever, or any other serious preventable disease.

To get the facts to the people is one of the definite tasks of each State department of health. This is being done:

a. Teaching the people by demonstration.—The sanitary inspector, on going into a new community, picks out a few typical cases and treats them as an object-lesson. He calls attention to the more striking symptoms present in these cases; he secures specimens of their stools and exhibits the hookworm eggs under the miscroscope; he administers treatment and later exhibits the parasites that have been expelled. The recovery which follows treatment and cure speaks its own message. These demonstrations are being multiplied by the physicians who are treating the disease. Thus from small and scattered centers to ever-widening circles the people are being reached by these tangible facts which they can see and understand.

b. Teaching the people by examinations made at the State laboratory.—The examinations being made at the State laboratory are demonstrating that the infection is widespread—much more so than any of us suspected one year ago. The infection has in this short time been demonstrated in 91 out of a total of 100 counties in Virginia; in 97 out of the 98 counties in North Carolina; in 22 out of 43 counties in South Carolina, and these distributed over the whole State; in 108 of the 145 counties in Georgia; in 63 of the 67 counties in Alabama; in Louisiana two months' work has demonstrated infection in 23 parishes; in Mississippi it has been demonstrated in 65 of the 76 counties; in Arkansas, in 20 counties in the southern part of the State, where the survey has been made by personal inspection with microscopic examination; in Tennessee, which has no State laboratory, microscopic examinations by the State director and his staff have demonstrated the infection in 52 of the 96 counties, and these situated in every section of the State.

These examinations being made at the laboratories are

showing also that very many people are infected. The North Carolina State laboratory has just completed an examination of 5,556 people, taken by groups without reference to clinical symptoms. These people are college students, soldiers, orphans, public-school children of all ages and conditions. The records show that of the 5,556 persons, 2,408, or 43 per cent, are infected.

These two groups of facts are growing in volume daily; being the records of microscopic examinations made by experts, their accuracy cannot be questioned. They show that the infection is very prevalent among the people. that all classes of people are subject to it, and that it is distributed over large areas of each of these States; they bring home to the people living in these infected areas the importance to the individual and to the community of having every carrier of infection examined and treated.

c. Teaching the people by examination of the school children.—The people are being led to seek examination and treatment by systematic examination of the children in the schools. The sanitary inspector reaches the schools of a county through the State superintendent of education, the county superintendent, the school boards, and principals. On going into a school he makes a clinical examination of all the children, keeping a record of those that show clinical symptoms of hookworm disease. For each of these, notice is sent to the parent and to the family physician, calling attention to the findings and advising that a specimen be submitted to the physician or to the State laboratory for microscopical examination. Many of the inspectors collect the specimens and send them to the laboratory. The parent is given the result of the microscopic examination, and, if it is positive, is urged to have the child treated by the family physician.

For demonstration and as a check to his own clinical diagnosis, the inspector collects specimens from all the children of a few schools and submits them to the laboratory for examination.

Teachers are becoming active in this work; some of them are becoming expert in recognizing the symptoms of the disease, and urge parents of children showing these symptoms to have them examined. An instructor in one State normal school has examined a large group of student teachers in the institution and is teaching them how to recognize the clinical symptoms and to make the microscopic diagnosis— this with a view to their being able to protect the children in their own schools and to aid in stamping out this disease in the communities to which they may be called as teachers. The teacher thus trained will be the physician's best ally in the work.

d. Teaching the people by example.—The people are being led to seek examination and treatment by the coöperation of public-spirited, influential citizens. The inspectors, on going into a new community, frequently have the coöperation of a group of leading citizens, who ask to be examined and who let the fact be noised abroad. In one State a group of 600 college men submitted to examination and pledged themselves to use their influence each in his own community to get others to be examined and treated. The State universities and a few other colleges of North Carolina, South Carolina, and Mississippi have given their active coöperation and have made their influence felt throughout their respective States.

e. Teaching the people by means of public lectures and the printed page.—In each State the State board of health is disseminating these facts and enlarging the sphere of these influences by means of public lectures and the printed page. The State director and his staff make it a part of the work to give illustrated lectures to teachers, schools, and citizen audiences. In these lectures they use charts, photographs, and lantern slides and supplement these with facts gathered from the whole experience to show as concretely as possible what hookworm disease means to the people of that State in terms of economic loss and human suffering and inefficiency.

In each of the States the State board of health has issued one or more special bulletins showing the effects of the disease, and has distributed these broadcast. Some of the States are distributing in even larger numbers a small folder setting forth in simple language the essential points and giving directions for sending specimens to the State laboratory for free examination. Teachers, physicians, and traveling men are distributing this literature. A physician in Alabama recently reported that he takes a supply of one bulletin with him on every trip into the country. When he meets a child showing symptoms of the disease he hands him a copy, saying, "Show this to your mother and tell her I say I think you have that disease, and that you ought to see your family physician."

The State directors in Virginia, North Carolina, and Mississippi have the public press work well organized and are making systematic use of the county papers as an agency for getting the facts out to the people.

That the people are responding to these efforts is indicated by this record of examinations for hookworm disease made at the North Carolina State laboratory:

Examinations for quarter ending Mar. 31, 1910.... 70
" " " " June 30, 1910.... 486
" " " " Sept. 30, 1910.... 2,421
" " " " Dec. 31, 1911.... 4,972

(3) **Providing for the treatment of the indigent.**—Very many of the sufferers from hookworm disease, on account of extreme poverty, are not able to pay for treatment or even for the necessary medicine; and these as a rule are the more severe cases, for poverty is one of the distressing results of the disease. It works slowly through a long series of years, sapping the vitality and thereby destroying the earning power of its victims. Many families in heavily infected areas have never been free from the disease, and are today suffering the cumulative results of conditions that have come down even from preceding generations. To provide for the treatment of these is one of the most stubborn practical problems that the directors of the work are having to meet.

The Florida State board of health is meeting it by paying to the physicians of the State three dollars a case for all cases cured. This payment is made from the public-health fund of the State. The Florida board can do this; its public-health fund is on a mill basis and amounts to about $75,000 a year. This is not possible with present funds in any other State. In Virginia some voluntary organizations have been formed to raise funds for this purpose. In North Carolina and Virginia the physicians in many counties have agreed by formal resolution to prescribe for hookworm disease free to the poor, and the women's betterment associations in these counties in North Carolina have agreed to supply the funds for the medicine. Cotton-mill owners in some cases and in others public-spirited citizens have provided medicine for the indigent. In Arkansas, county organizations formed for the eradication of hookworm disease undertake to provide for treatment of all who need the aid. All these efforts help; but these agencies are not permanent and cannot of themselves meet the situation.

In Mississippi a free dispensary has been opened at Columbia for the treatment of hookworm disease in Marion county. The county board of supervisors recently made an appropriation from the county funds for the purpose of supplying the drugs; the county health officer provided four rooms with hall and lavatory; the Commercial Club of Columbia supplied the rooms with beds; the local physicians offered coöperation in giving treatment. The dispensary is running at its full capacity and hundreds are being turned away for lack of facilities. This is the most promising move that has been made in the direction of supplying treatment for the indigent.

(4) **Results.**—For summary of activities and results see Tables 1 and 2.

a. Table 1 shows the number of physicians in the State; what has been done to enlist them in the work; the estimated number treating the disease. The physician once enlisted is in the work for life.

b. Table 2 shows examinations made and cases treated. By devoting itself directly to the treatment of cases the State organizations could have made a definite record of a much larger number of cases treated; enlisting physicians now insures for the future multiplication of results.

c. The largest result achieved this year does not appear in the tables, namely, public sentiment created.

3. **Putting a stop to soil pollution.**—The final task in this work is to stamp out hookworm infection by putting a stop to soil pollution. The work is one of education and will require years for its accomplishment. Two lines of work are now in progress:

(1) **Sanitary survey.**—The State organization is conducting a sanitary survey to determine the existing conditions responsible for the presence and spread of the disease. The sanitary inspectors are supplied with forms on which they report the sanitary conditions surrounding homes, churches, schools, saw-mills, and similar industrial plants.

In these nine States is a population of 17,743,253, distributed over an area of 415,950 square miles. About 80 per cent of these people live in the open country, where since the earliest settlement soil pollution has been almost universal and with no thought of its serious consequences. (See Table 3.)

(2) **Teaching the people the dangers of soil pollution and how to stop it.**—To get fourteen millions of people, distributed over half a million square miles of territory, to abandon a habit ingrained by centuries of usage and to conform to specific sanitary regulation will require the coöperation of permanent agencies in a system of education directed definitely to this end and kept up for a long period of time. A beginning has been made.

a. Teaching the people by public lectures.—The State

director of sanitation and each member of his staff is supplied with lantern and a set of slides. Each man is now making his own photographs of local conditions. Some of the inspectors are preparing a series of charts. With this equipment they are perpared to tell and illustrate the life story of the parasite; to show how the young hookworms get into the soil and under what conditions they thrive there; to make vivid by pictures how the infection is spread when the barefoot child walks over this ground; to show how soil pollution may be prevented; to intensify the lesson by exhibiting photographs of local conditions.

The inspector tells this story to popular audiences in the evenings, and to the schools which he inspects during the day. One inspector says his purpose is to make the story so simple, so direct, so vivid that every child will feel it tingle on the bottom of his bare foot when he walks on polluted soil.

This story has been told 1,240 times during the year by the regular staff in these nine States; it has reached more than 196,000 people. The school child has repeated it at home and neighbor has repeated it to neighbor.

b. Teaching the people by means of bulletins and folders.—The State boards of health in these nine States have published and distributed during the year 546,000 copies of special bulletins and folders on the dangers of soil pollution and how to avoid them. (See Table 4a.)

c. Teaching the people through the public press.—The State director and his staff make it a part of the work to visit the papers of the State to establish personal relations with the editor, to give him first-hand knowledge of the facts, and to enlist the paper as a permanent agency in the service. Virginia, North Carolina, and Mississippi have the coöperation of practically the entire State press and have the press service effectively organized. Definite organization of this service in each State will be effected as soon as practicable. (See Table 4a.)

d. *Teaching the people through the schools.*—The work of enlisting the schools as a permanent agency in this sanitary service has only begun. The State superintendent of education in each State has offered his active coöperation. Three lines of definite work are now in progress:

(a) *Putting a stop to soil pollution at the schools.*— For the protection of the children and as an object-lesson to the community, sanitary privies are being built at the schools. This is being urged by the sanitary inspectors in all the States, by the State organizer of school improvement leagues in all the States except North Carolina, and by many of the county superintendents. In Virginia and Louisiana the State boards of health have promulgated regulations having the force of law requiring that all the schools of those States be provided with sanitary toilets; the State departments of education agree to coöperate in carrying them into effect. The work has been done in two districts in Virginia and is under way in 24 other districts. The county school boards of four counties in North Carolina and one county in Tennessee have ordered that sanitary privies be provided at all the schools in these counties, and that the expense be borne by the county school funds. Virginia has a record of 1,570 privies built. This work will be pushed systematically.

(b) *Teaching the school children the dangers of soil pollution and how to avoid them.*—The sanitary inspector, after inspecting the children in a school, gives them definite instruction in sanitary measures. In some communities physicians have volunteered to give this instruction at the schools. In two towns in North Carolina and two counties in Georgia the school authorities have provided local funds for this service. The Mississippi State board of health has issued a bulletin on hookworm disease especially designed for use in the schools; it has also supplied the schools with a placard to be framed and hung where it can be easily read. The North Carolina State department of education has published a fifty-thousand edition of a bulletin on soil pollution for use in the public schools of the State. This has been distributed through the county superintendents to the public-school teachers with instructions that it be used as the basis of instruction to the school children. Dr. Ferrell, the State director of sanitation in that State, recently prepared for the department of education an outline for a series of talks on hookworm disease and soil pollution, the outline to be published by the department of education and distributed to the teachers for use as a basis for oral instruction to the children in all the public schools of the State.

The Arkansas State department of education has a bulletin ready for publication. In the State Normal School, at Athens, Georgia, the student teachers are being given instruction in hookworm disease to the end that they as teachers may be able to give definite instruction to the children in their own schools.

These are permanent educational agencies; the work which this year has made only a beginning will go on increasing in volume and efficiency.

IV. Summary of expenditures.—

	Expended by—		
	State.	Commission.	Total.
Alabama	$150.00	$1,444.32	$1,594.32
Arkansas		4,474.20	4,474.20
Georgia	1,880.00	6,933.86	8,813.86
Louisiana	400.00	549.99	949.99
Mississippi	4,500.00	6,283.11	10,783.11
North Carolina	2,000.00	9,948.76	11,948.76
South Carolina	1,000.00	4,029.91	5,029.91
Tennessee	692.86	5,002.20	5,695.06
Virginia	2,630.00	8,353.09	10,983.09
Totals	$13,252.86	$47,019.44	$60,272.30

Enlisting the Physicians.

State.	Number of physicians in State.	Number of physicians personally instructed.	Number of lectures given to physicians.	Number of physicians reached.	Number of letters and circulars sent to physicians.	Number of bulletins sent to physicians.	Physicians now treating the disease.
Alabama	2,200	115*	5	85	....	2,200	440*
Arkansas	3,600	275	21	450	3,000	7,000	500*
Georgia	2,887	800*	9	156	2,887	2,887	576
Louisiana	2,033	359	3	165	2,500*	7,000	
Mississippi	2,054	280	10	200	2,454	4,168	450
North Carolina	1,500	674	18	745	3,418	4,000	838
South Carolina	1,113	84	9	350*	1,113	1,113	100
Tennessee	3,449	400*	14	250*	1,200*	6,898	
Virginia	2,300	461	45	1,200*	....	13,800	500*

* Estimated.

Examinations and Treatment.

State.	Number of schools inspected.	Number of farms or families examined.	Number of persons examined.	Positive diagnoses. Clinical.	Positive diagnoses. Microscopic.	Persons treated. On record.	Persons treated. Estimated. Not on record.	Total.
Alabama	31	....	1,262	801	92	3,330	....	3,330
Arkansas	46	450	2,250	1,387	442	1,400	6,000	7,400
Georgia	163	240*	17,775	4,572*	1,165	....	....	....
Louisiana	79	240*	5,000*	1,000*	79	....	....	....
Mississippi	150*	472	9,331	2,737	1,682	824	4,000	4,824
North Carolina	238	390*	33,162	4,408	7,949	8,000	6,000	14,000
South Carolina	115	200	4,900	2,200	85	665	400	1,065
Tennessee	136	1,564	3,055	1,052	545	204	....	204
Virginia	300*	2,500*	25,000*	10,000*	2,750	....	8,000	8,000

* Estimated.

Putting a Stop to Soil Pollution—Results of Sanitary Survey.

State.	Area (sq. miles).	Population.	Per cent living in country.	Sanitary conditions.
Alabama.........	51,000	2,138,000	70	Of 31 schools inspected, only 1 in 5 has privy of any kind for girls, and but 1 in 10 has privy of any kind for boys.
Arkansas.........	53,045	1,500,000	80	Inspection of schools, churches, farms, and saw-mills has failed thus far to discover one sanitary privy outside of cities and towns.
Georgia..........	58,980	2,609,000	83	Of homes, schools, and churches outside of cities, majority have no privy of any kind; sanitary privies very rare.
Louisiana........	48,506	1,656,388	63	Open earth closets practically universal.
Mississippi.......	46,340	1,708,272	80	Relatively few homes and schools in the country have closets.
North Carolina...	52,000	2,246,000	82	Of 238 white schools inspected, only 6 have sanitary privies. Of 20 negro schools inspected, not one has sanitary privy. Mills inspected, 14; operatives, 5,700; open privies, 945; sanitary privies, 0.
South Carolina...	30,170	1,515,400	80	Fifty per cent of homes in rural districts have no closets. Fifty per cent of schools have no closets. Churches no toilets. Very few sanitary closets.
Tennessee........	42,050	2,185,789	80	Of 456 homes inspected, none have sanitary privies and only 285 have privies of any kind. At country homes, schools, churches, and saw-mills, privies of any sort reported exceptional.
Virginia..........	40,125	1,854,184	83.5	From a record of 1,000 farms inspected, only 15 per cent were using a privy of any kind. Of 7,088 schools in the State, only 3,830 have privy of any kind.

Putting a Stop to Soil Pollution—Educating the People.

State.	Through bulletins. Number of bulletins and leaflets distributed.	Through the press. Papers in State.	Number personally visited.	Letters to press.	Articles furnished for publication.	Attitude of press.
Alabama.......	20,000	247	10	23	19	In thorough sympathy.
Arkansas.......	60,000	210	65	420	12	Without exception favorable and willing to coöperate.
Georgia........	34,000	246	83	"Many."	150*	Cannot answer.
Louisiana......	25,000	78	20	128	3	Interested and ready to coöperate.
Mississippi....	65,000	130*	35	135	40*	At beginning indifferent; slight opposition. At present all papers coöperating.
North Carolina.	152,000	312	157*	1,248	305	At beginning indifferent, humorous, often resentful. Now not one opposing. Practically all give active coöperation.
South Carolina.	10,000	...	...	None.	50	Most of the papers are supporting the work.
Tennessee	70,000	...	30*	....	15*	Lukewarm.
Virginia........	110,000	150	25	300	1 each week.	Hopeful from start.

* Estimated.

THE ERADICATION OF HOOKWORM DISEASE.

Putting a Stop to Soil Pollution—Educating the People.

State.	Number of teachers in State.	Through the schools.				Through public lectures.	
		Teachers reached.					
		By visit.	By letter.	By bulletin or leaflet.	At institutes.	Number of lectures given.	Estimated number of persons reached by these lectures.	Sanitary privies built.

State.	Number of teachers in State.	By visit.	By letter.	By bulletin or leaflet.	At institutes.	Number of lectures given.	Estimated number of persons reached by these lectures.	Sanitary privies built.
Alabama	8,677	35	57	104	0	52	3,000	No report.
Arkansas	9,522	98	3,000	9,000	1,300*	58	30,000	
Georgia	.....	578*	600*	600*	Indefinite.	200*	17,000	
Louisiana	3,000*	800*	500*	All.	600*	171	21,000	
Mississippi	6,929	450	800	All.	3,500	254	35,000	75*
North Carolina	11,500	550	4,000	10,000	7,655	100	50,000	75
South Carolina	.....	800	50	1,000	300	75	6,000	No report.
Tennessee	10,400	No record.	No record.	All.	800*	65*	9,000	10
Virginia	8,407	1,100	All.	All.	5,000*	265	25,000	1,570

* Estimated

KEY, Maps 1 to 8.

○ Survey made in detail, infection HEAVY.
★ "   "   "   "   "   LIGHT.
★ Preliminary survey made, infection demonstrated.

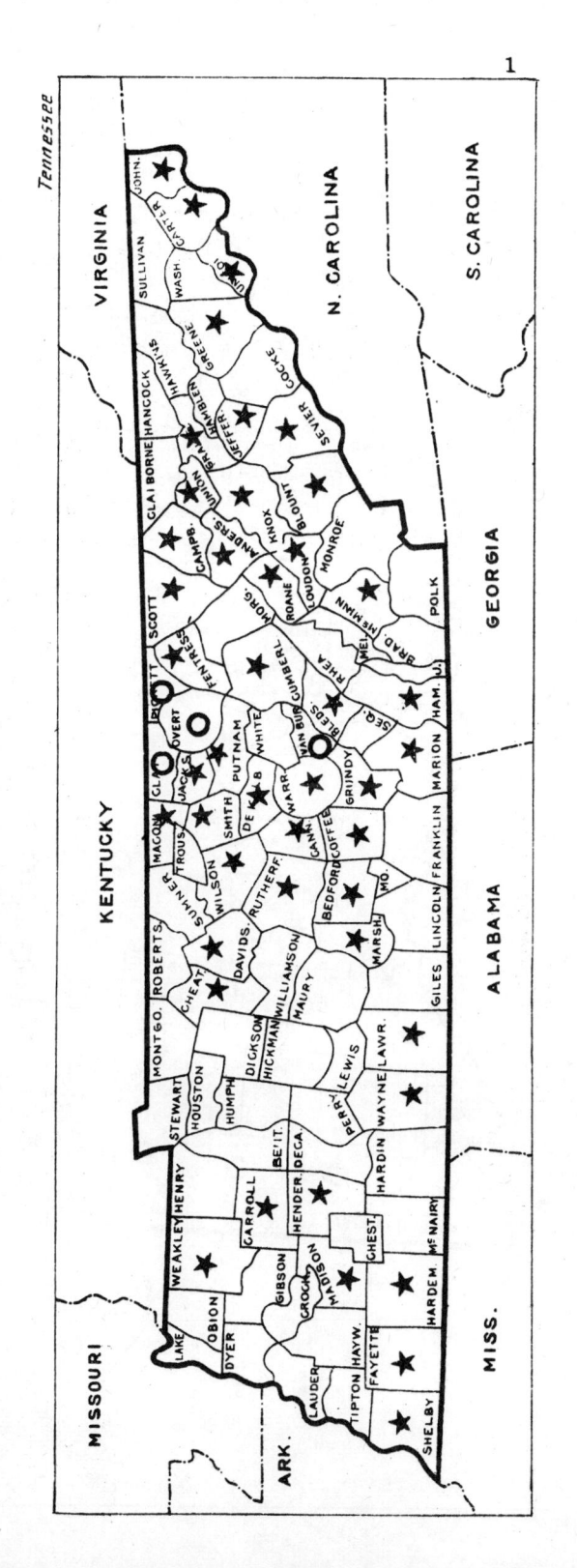

Mississippi

Alabama 3

4

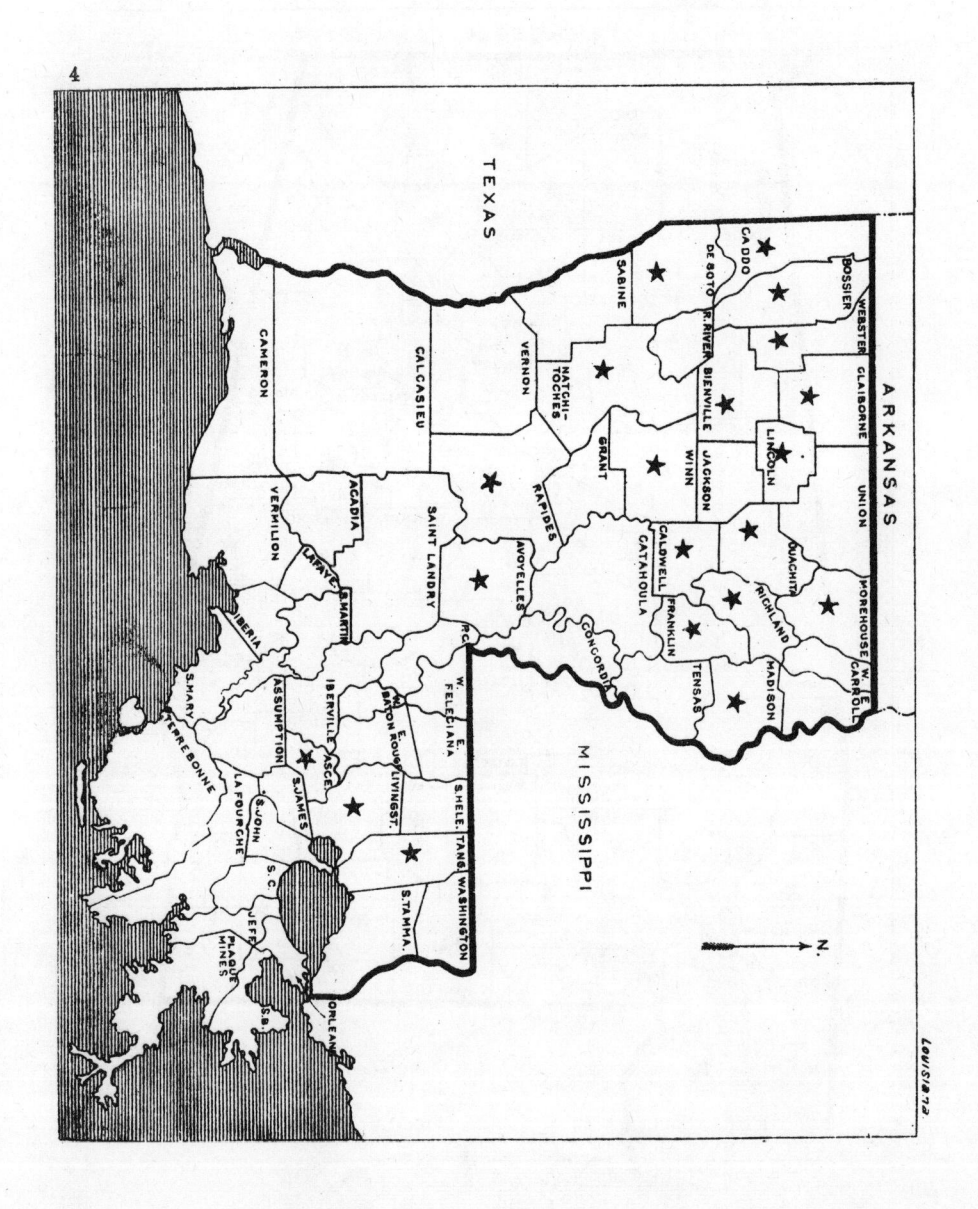

South Carolina

6   Georgia

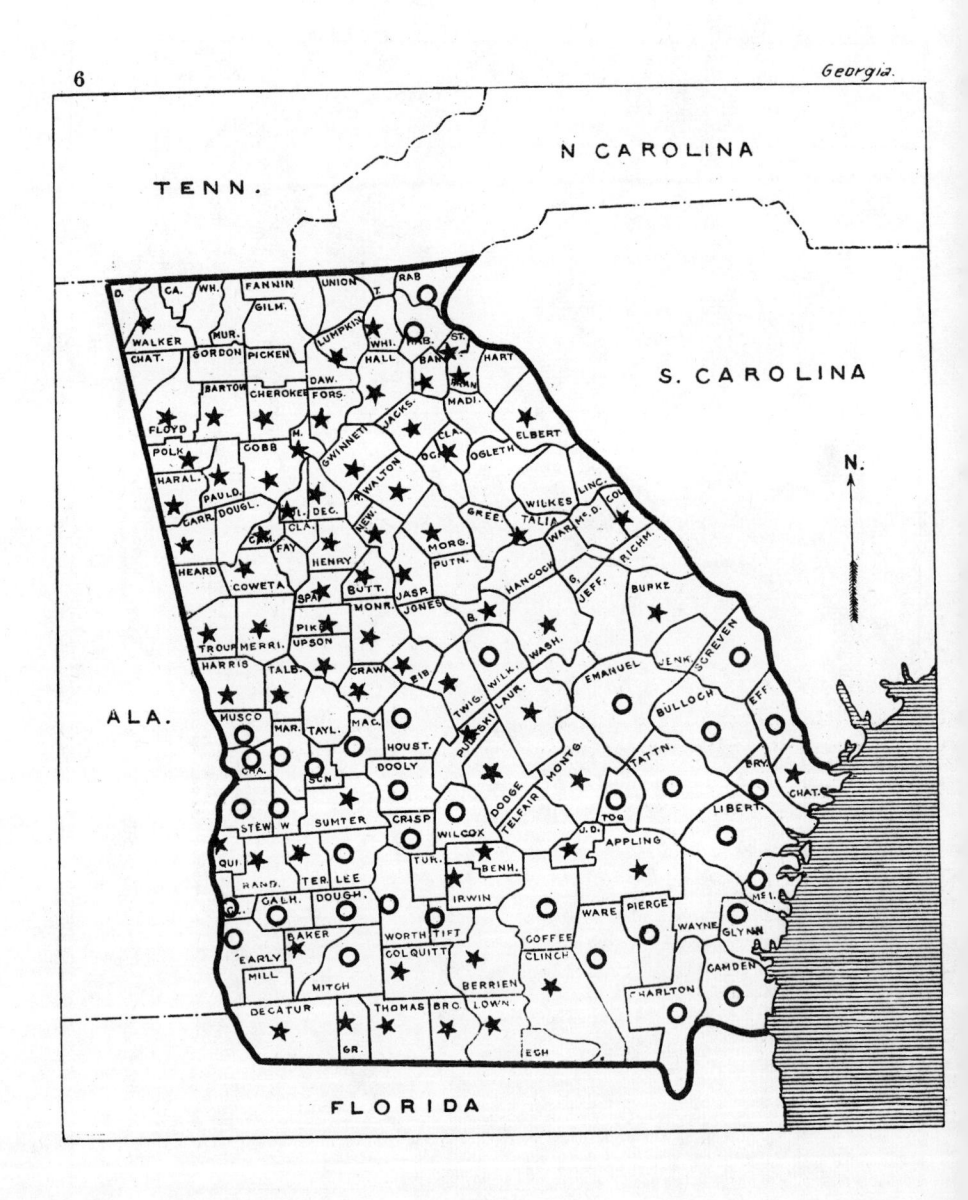

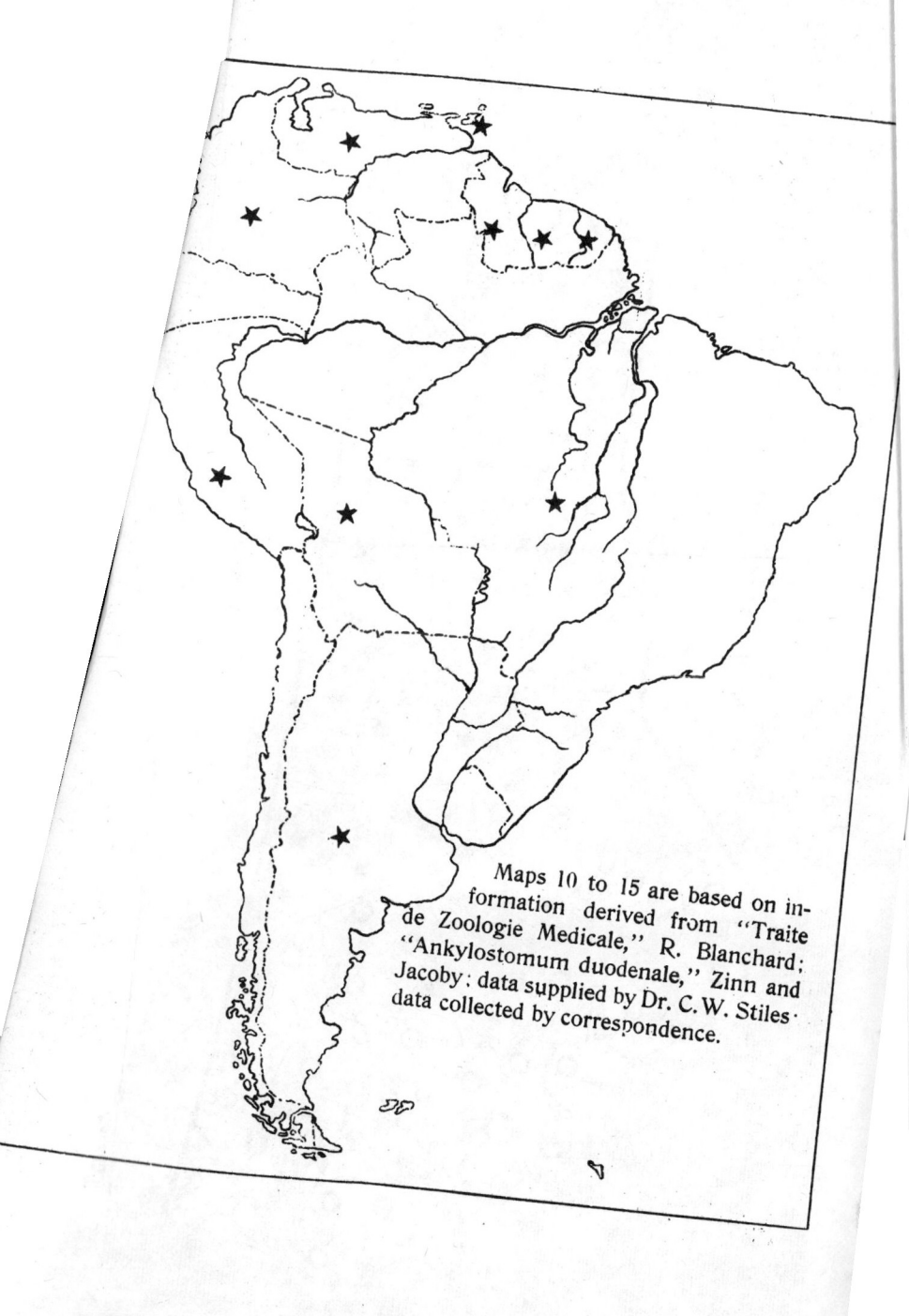

Maps 10 to 15 are based on information derived from "Traite de Zoologie Medicale," R. Blanchard; "Ankylostomum duodenale," Zinn and Jacoby; data supplied by Dr. C. W. Stiles; data collected by correspondence.

Arkansas.

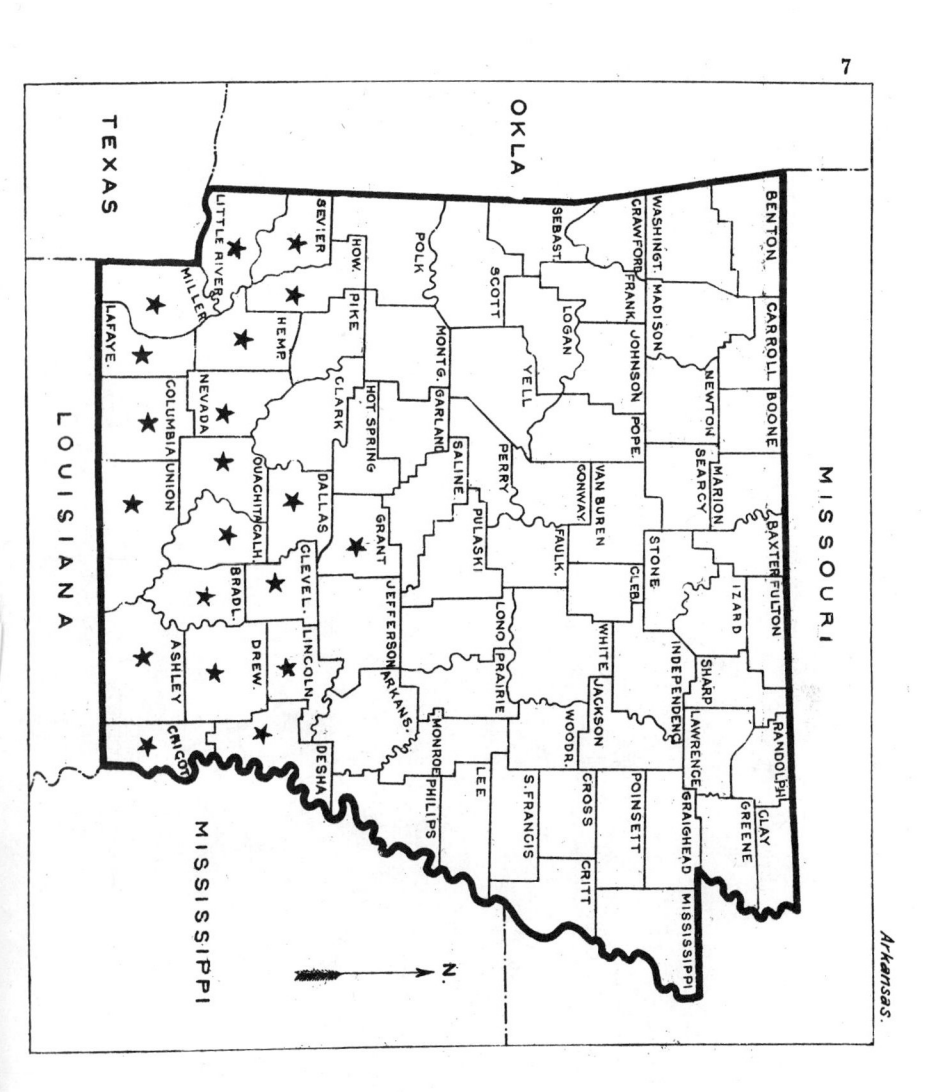

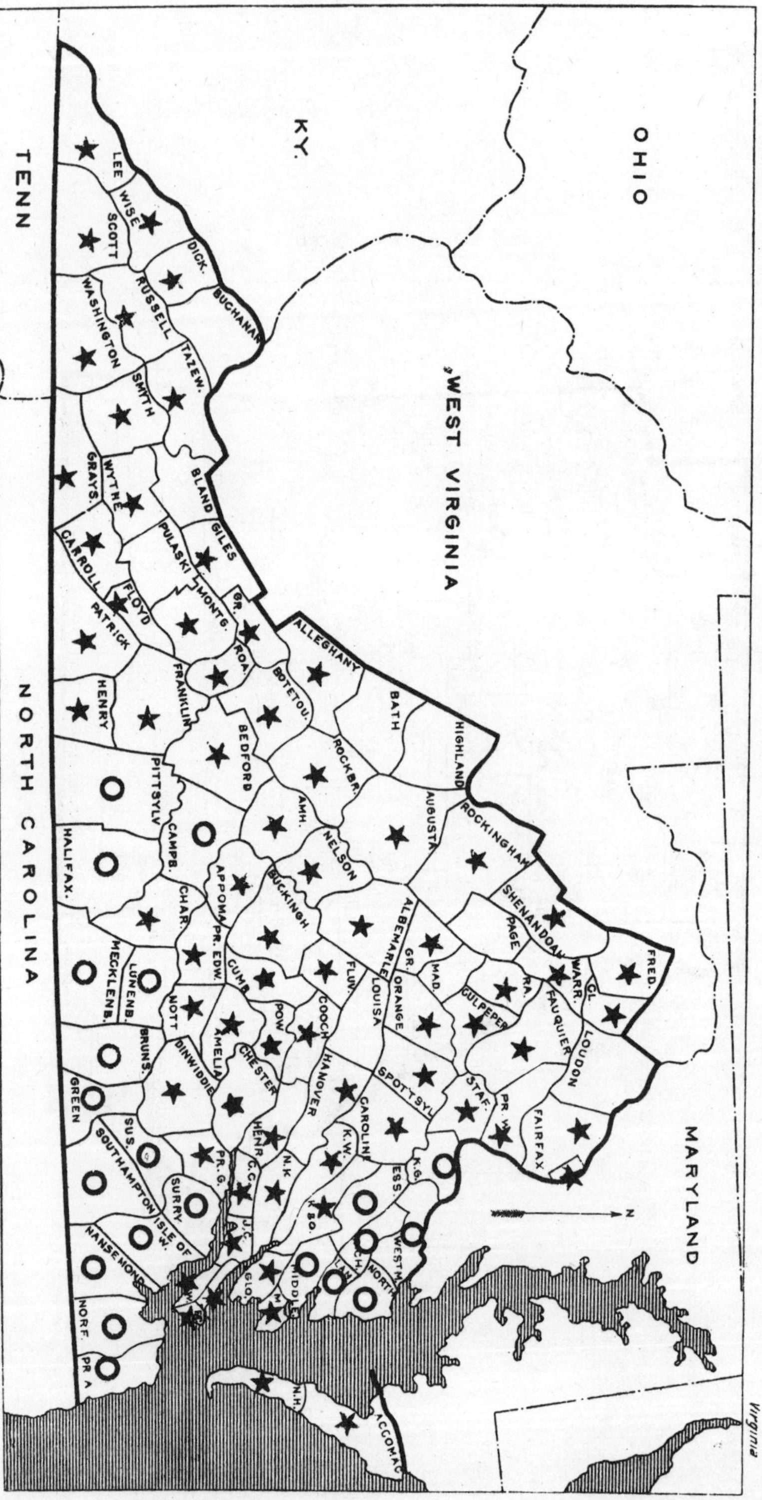

OHIO
KY.
TENN
WEST VIRGINIA
NORTH CAROLINA
MARYLAND
N
LEE
WISE
SCOTT
DICK.
BUCHANAN
RUSSELL
WASHINGTON
TAZEW.
SMITH
BLAND
WYTHE
GRAYS.
GILES
PULASKI
CARROLL
FLOYD
MONTG.
GR.
PATRICK
ROA.
ALLEGHANY
FRANKLIN
HENRY
BOTETOU.
BATH
HIGHLAND
BEDFORD
ROCKBR.
PITTSYLV.
CAMPB.
AMH.
AUGUSTA
ROCKINGHAM
NELSON
HALIFAX.
APPOMA.
CHAR.
BUCKINGH.
ALBEMARLE
SHENANDOAH
PAGE
PR. EDW.
CUMB.
FLUV.
GR.
MAD.
RA.
WARR.
CL.
FRED.
MECKLENB.
LUNENB.
NOTT.
AMELIA
POW.
COOCH.
LOUISA
ORANGE
CULPEPER
FAUQUIER
LOUDON
BRUNS.
DINWIDDIE
CHESTER
HANOVER
SPOTTSYL.
STAF.
PR. W.
FAIRFAX
GREEN
SUS.
SOUTHAMPTON
SURRY
PR. G.
HENR.
N.K.
CAROLINE
K.W.
K.G.
ESS.
C.C.
J.C.
K.BO.
WESTM.
NORTH
LAN.
RICH.
ISLE OF W.
NANSEMOND
GLO.
MIDDLE.
M.
NORF.
PR. A.
N.H.
ACCOMAC

10

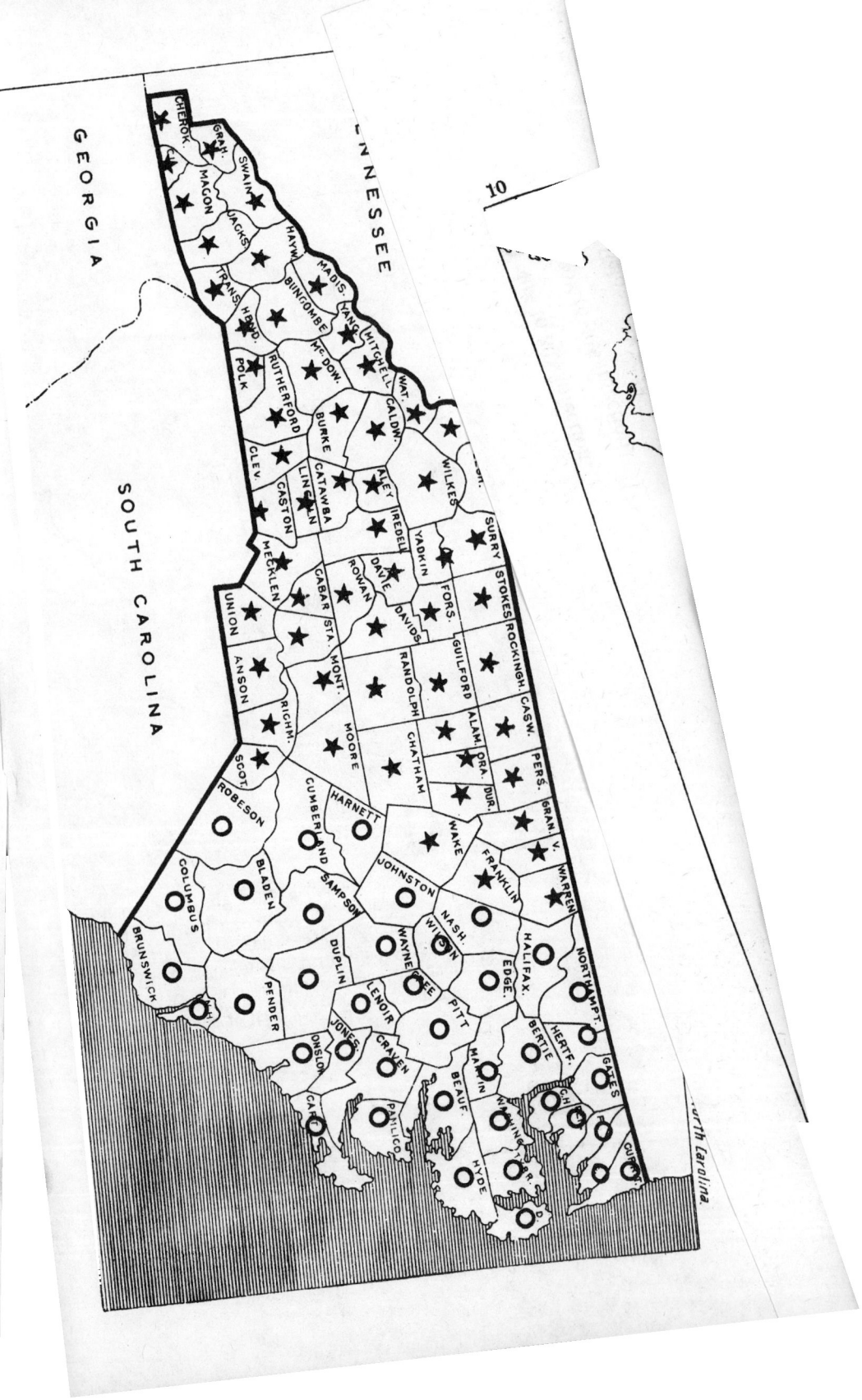

11

12

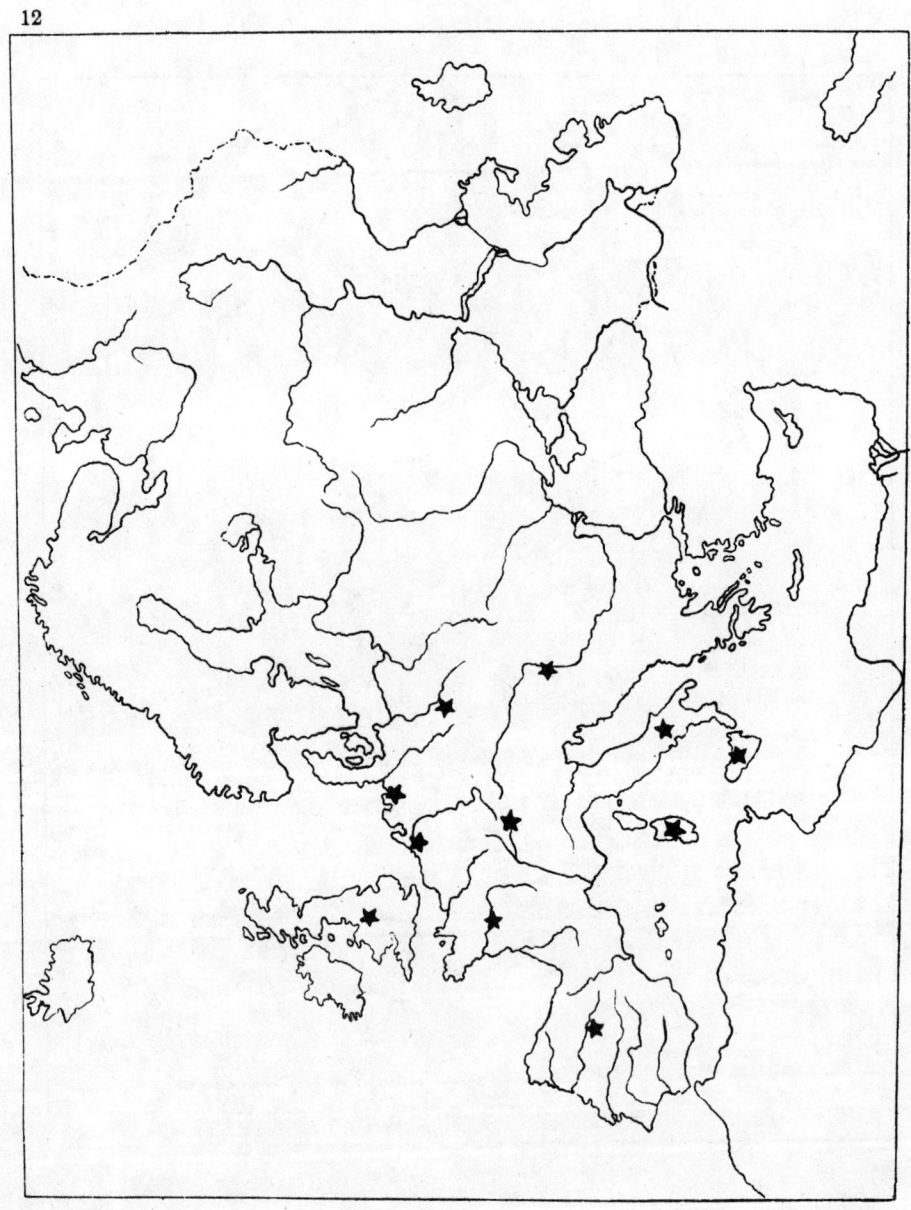

13

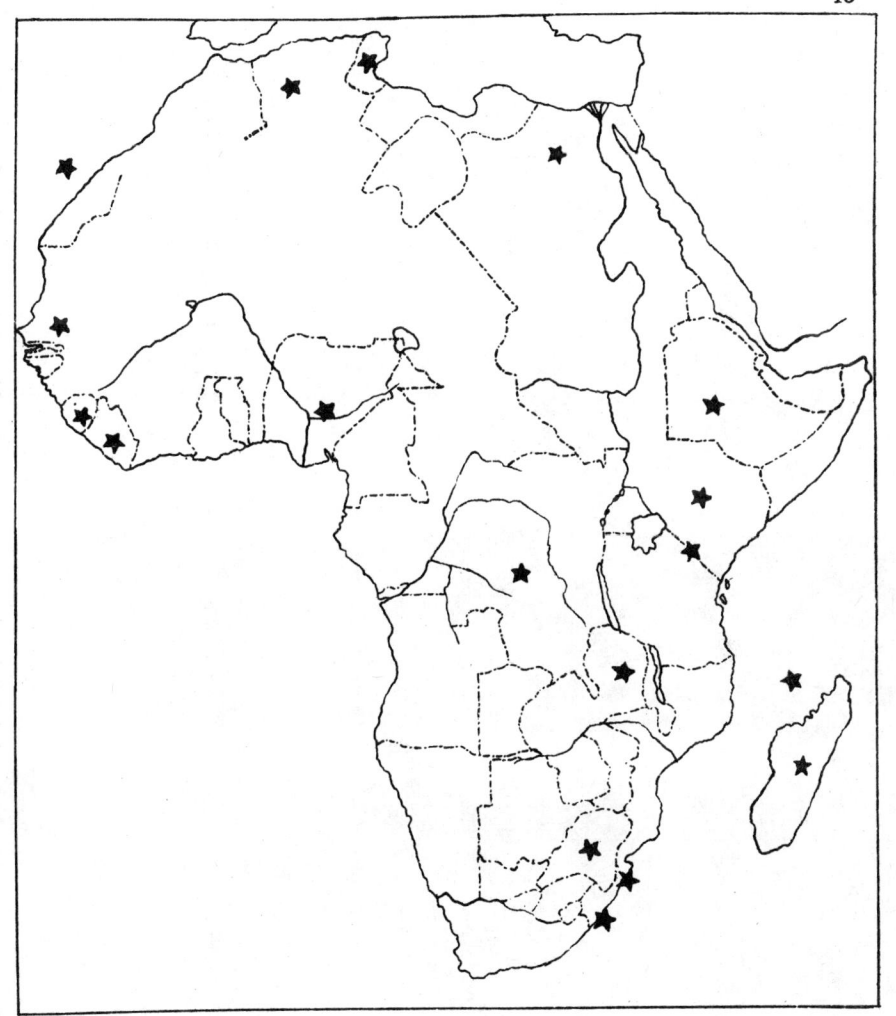

14

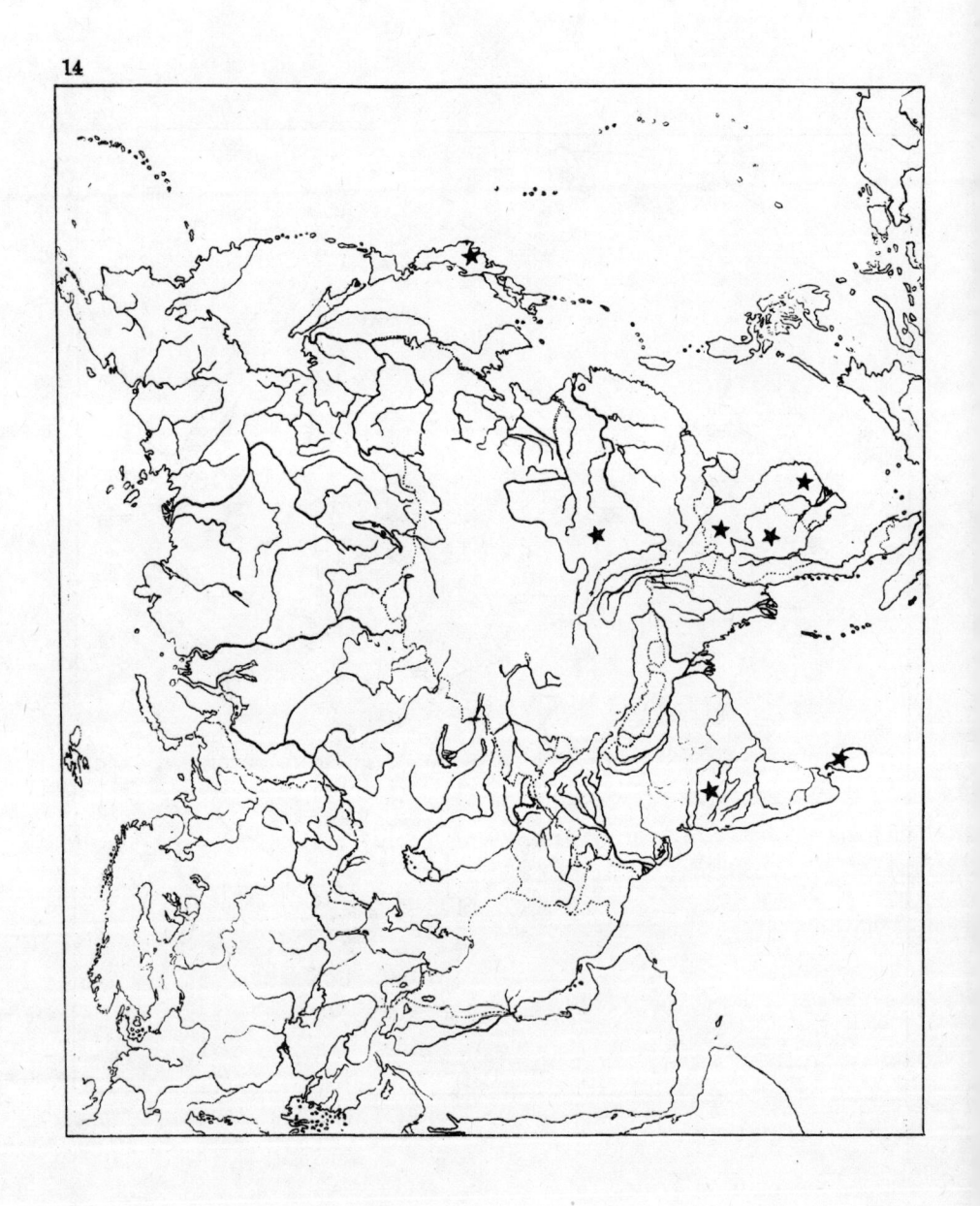

15

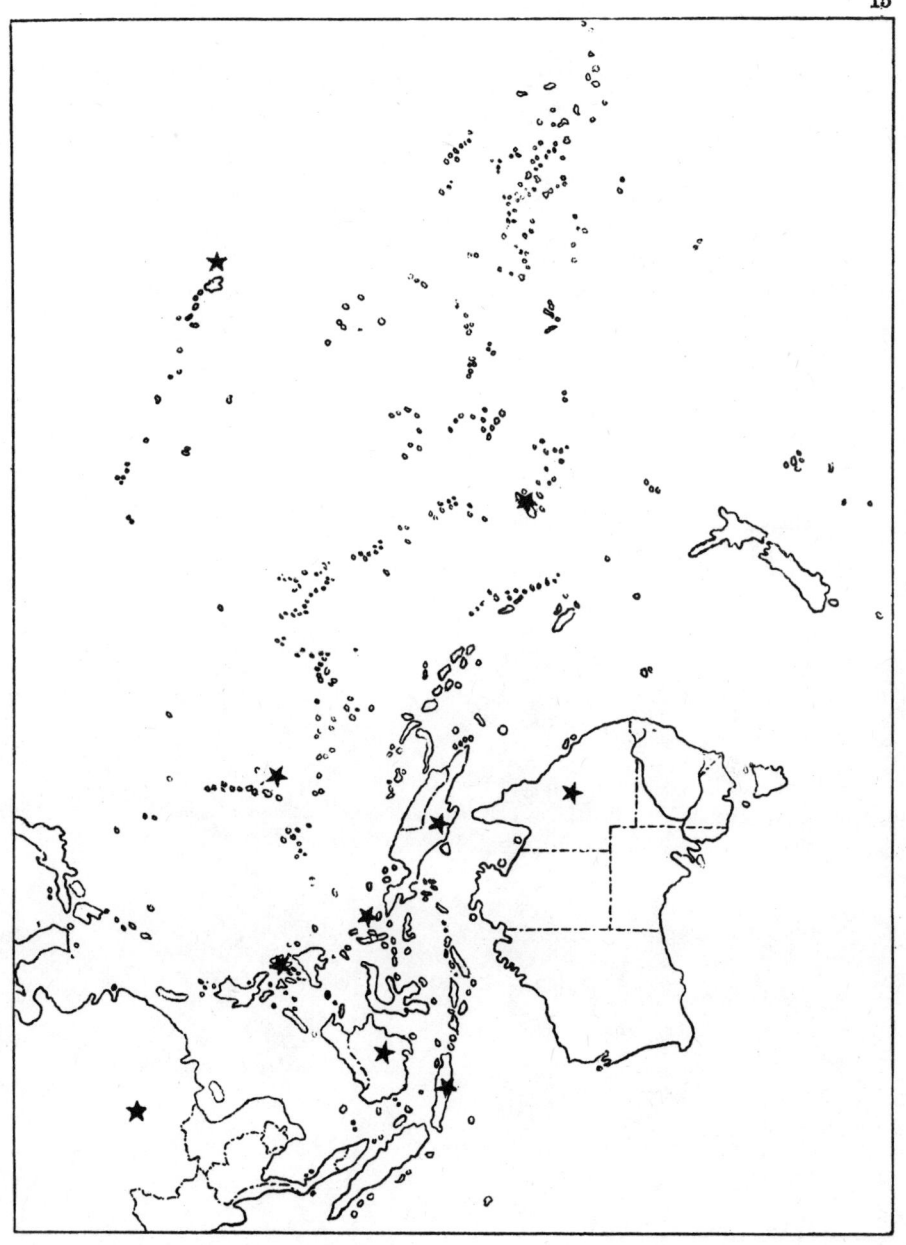

APPENDIX.

The Florida State Department of Health had instituted a campaign against hookworm disease before the Rockefeller Sanitary Commission was organized. In response to Dr. J. Y. Porter's very cordial invitation, the administrative secretary of the Commission and many of the State directors of sanitation visited Florida early in the year to study the methods and results of that work. Not only are we personally indebted to Dr. Porter and his staff for many courtesies, but to them the service is indebted for cordial cooperation and helpful suggestion at every point. We have asked the privilege of appending this summary of the work in Florida for its intrinsic merit and as an acknowledgment of our indebtedness to the work and workers in that State.

FLORIDA STATE BOARD OF HEALTH.

A Summary of Hookworm Work Accomplished in Florida from October 12, 1909, to December 31, 1910.

MILEAGE.

The State health officer and three assistant State health officers during this period, in travel chargeable to hookworm disease, covered—

By railway	6,220 miles
By teams	1,070 miles
By boats	330 miles
A total of	7,620 miles

EXPENSES INCURRED.

Salaries of two assistant State health officers while actively engaged in the hookworm campaign	$1,508.30
Travel expenses during the same period (an average per man per month of $97)	1,057.15
Total expended by the two field men...	$2,565.45
Cost of hookworm literature during 1909 and 1910, which includes circular letters, case record blanks, and 20,000 leaflets for popular distribution	65.00
Cost of that portion of Florida Health Notes, the monthly bulletin, devoted to hookworm disease, being 72 pages, or 4½ monthly issues of 16 pages, with a circulation per month of 17,000, and equivalent to 1,224,000 pages....	592.00
Laboratory salaries and maintenance, 1909, chargeable	525.00
Laboratory salaries and maintenance, 1910, chargeable	2,650.00
Six hundred and two indigent cases treated, treatment paid for by State board of health, at $3 each	1,806.00
Travel expenses of State health officer and assistant State Health Officer Byrd, in inspections, delivering lectures, etc.	534.00
Total expense	$8,737.45

Synopsis of the Work Accomplished by Two Assistant State Health Officers.

TIME ENGAGED.

October 12, 1909, to March 24, 1910	163 days
January 3, 1910, to May 11, 1910	128 days
August 28, 1910, to September 30, 1910	33 days
Number of days in the field	324

MILEAGE TRAVELED.

By rail	3,360 miles
By teams	1,070 miles
By boats	330 miles
Total	4,400 miles

Three thousand two hundred and twenty-seven suspicious cases of hookworm disease found.

MICROSCOPICAL EXAMINATIONS MADE.

Positive	399
Negative	179
Total	578

Inspected 79 white schools; 4 negro schools.
Visited 94 towns in 10 counties.

Lectures before public audiences	13
Lectures before school children	79
Lectures delivered by Dr. Byrd	14
Total	108

Other work accomplished during the same period:
Two outbreaks of scarlet fever directed.
Four conferences regarding disposal of city sewage.
Two smallpox cases isolated and cared for.
Two epidemics of typhoid fever investigated.
Prevalence of catarrhal and follicular conjunctivitis reported in five schools.

Record of Cases.

Under the plan of the State board of health to pay physicians three dollars for treatment of indigent cases of hookworm disease, 602 cases have, during the year 1910, been paid for.

Conforming to the minimum requirement of the board in the matter of treatment, 67.87 per cent of these 602 cases were cured. Twenty-three cases—3.8 per cent of the series—were also freed of the worms, the treatment progressing beyond the minimum requirement up to four, five, seven, and nine courses of treatment.

It is found that this plan has been taken advantage of by 45 physicians in 23 counties of the State.

The patients so treated were distributed over 78 towns in the 23 counties.

Hookworm Examinations Made in the Bacteriological Laboratories.

1904 to 1908, one laboratory.............. 507 specimens
1909, with one laboratory, 248 positive, 397
  negative, and 23 unfit for examination.... 668 specimens

In March, 1910, a bacteriological laboratory was established by the State board of health at Tampa, and in July, 1910, an additional laboratory was established in Pensacola, Fla. The central laboratory is located at Jacksonville.

During 1910 the three laboratories examined 16,095 disease specimens of all kinds. Of this number 45 per cent, or 7,402, have been examinations for the hookworm. Fifty-two per cent of the specimens of all kinds received at the Jacksonville laboratory were submitted for examination for hookworms; 28 per cent of the specimens received at the Tampa laboratory were for hookworm examination, and 33 per cent of those received at the Pensacola laboratory were for this examination.

Summary Examinations for Animal Parasites at the Three Laboratories, 1910.

HOOKWORMS.

	Positive.	Negative.	Unfit.	Total.
January............	210	151	12	373
February...........	205	165	2	372
March.............	446	293	0	739
April..............	362	262	8	632
May...............	424	348	19	791
June...............	309	295	11	615
July...............	415	311	8	734
August.............	430	341	8	779
September.........	454	393	2	849
October............	370	221	3	594
November..........	204	219	0	523
December..........	224	177	0	401
Total..........	4,153	3,176	73	7,402

Number of examinations for other parasites................ 308
Add to this the examination by two assistant { Positive, 399
State officers in the field................ { Negative, 179
                                                         ——
                                                         578

Total number of examinations.................... 8,288

Four thousand five hundred and fifty-two, or 61.49 per cent, of the above examinations were positive for hookworms.

The examinations for parasites other than the hookworm were divided as follows:

Amœba coli	2
Ascaris lumbricoides	73
Lamblia intestinalis	1
Oxyuris vermicularis	19
Strongyloides intestinalis	8
Tapeworms	95
Trichocephalus dispar	106
Unidentified eggs	4
Total	308

Of these 308 specimens, 67 were examined in the field by two assistant State health officers, and 241 were examined by two of the laboratories.

During 1910 the laboratory at Jacksonville has sent out in the State 10,004 containers for submitting specimens for examination for hookworm disease, 12 per cent of which have not been returned.

During 1910 specimens of all kinds were received from 562 physicians in 197 towns, distributed among all of the 47 counties.

During 1910 specimens have been received from 34 towns in which no physician lives. These 34 towns are distributed over 17 counties.

One thousand physicians are licensed to practice in Florida. Specimens of all kinds have been received from a little more than 50 per cent of them.

Results of the Campaign.

An attempt was made to determine the number of cases of hookworm disease treated in five counties which had, six months before, been thoroughly gone over in the campaign by the assistant State health officers. This territory was canvassed again, and every physician interviewed and information obtained as to the number of cases he had treated. It was found that 66 physicians in 24 towns had treated 3,142 cases.

Extending the investigation, it was found that 562 physicians, in 197 towns distributed over the 47 counties, had submitted specimens of all kinds to the laboratories for examination during 1910. Two hundred and one of these physicians in 39 towns did not, however, submit hookworm specimens; but 58 of these 201 physicians, it is known, and who live in 33 towns, are treating hookworm disease. Among these 58 physicians are many of the pioneers in this work, who use their own microscope for diagnostic purposes.

Assuming that the physicians interviewed represent an average, then the 419 physicians, it will be seen, have treated 20,000 cases, 60 per cent of which were cured. This does not account for the other 500 physicians in Florida who have not submitted specimens to the laboratories, but many of whom, if not all, have been treating the disease.

Quite recently a map of Florida was taken, and with the Medical Directory of the American Medical Association and office records of the board as guides, a tack was placed at every town where there is one or more physicians. At such towns as it was known that hookworm disease was being treated, a black-headed tack was placed. At other places a red-headed tack was placed. It is found that the black-headed tacks are far in the ascendency, and that as our informtion becomes more and more complete the red-headed tacks are often disappearing from the map. It is believed at the present time that there is hardly a physician in the State not treating hookworm disease. This belief is based upon the fact that for the last several months not one such has been encountered, notwithstanding a corps of four or five physicians have been covering the State in all directions.

It may be said at this juncture that the hookworm work in Florida would continue to go on, even though the board took no further part in it; that the hookworm problem will now．solve itself, so far as it can be solved; that people in all walks of life, when indisposed from any cause they do not understand, suspect hookworms, and have examinations made accordingly; that hookworm information is now household information, and these things, after all, are the most that can be hoped for in this generation.

It is the intention of the board to continue payment for the treatment of indigent cases and to continue publishing literature on hookworm disease, to continue the educational crusade, but it believes that the great mass of the important work in this direction is behind rather than ahead.

PELLAGRA CAUSATION AND A METHOD OF PREVENTION

Joseph Goldberger

PELLAGRA: CAUSATION AND A METHOD OF PREVENTION

A SUMMARY OF SOME OF THE RECENT STUDIES OF THE UNITED STATES PUBLIC HEALTH SERVICE

JOSEPH GOLDBERGER, M.D.
Surgeon, U. S. Public Health Service

WASHINGTON, D. C.

One of the outstanding features of the epidemiology of pellagra is the striking relation of the disease to poverty. In reflecting on this and in considering the elements that differentiate poverty from affluence, diet, in view of the conspicuous place it has always had in discussions of the disease, naturally arrested attention. Approaching the problem of the possible relation of diet to pellagra in this way, it seemed permissible to assume, on the one hand, that the diet of the poor, that is, of those who as a class are the principal sufferers from the disease, is, for some reason, pellagra-producing, and, on the other, that the diet of the well-to-do, who, as a class, are practically exempt, is, for some reason, pellagra-preventing. The thought was near, therefore, that it might be possible to prevent the disease by providing those subject to pellagra with a diet such as that enjoyed by well-to-do people. Early in 1914, it was proposed to put this idea to a practical test.

Before the test was actually begun, studies of the prevalence of pellagra at institutions, such as prisons, asylums and orphanages, were made, the results of which, in the light of the recent advances in our knowledge of beriberi, very strongly suggested the idea that the disease was dependent on a diet that was, for some reason, faulty, and that this fault was in some way either prevented or corrected by including in the diet suitable proportions of the fresh animal protein foods

---

10. Typhoid in the Large Cities of the United States in 1914, special article, THE JOURNAL A. M. A., April 17, 1915, p. 1322.

and legumes.[1] These findings not only confirmed the original conception, but also helped in defining this more clearly, and, moreover, made it possible to formulate more definite plans, which were temporarily broadened to include a test of diet in the treatment as well as in the prevention of the disease.

TREATMENT

At my suggestion, Dr. W. F. Lorenz,[2] who was at that time studying the psychiatric manifestations of pellagra at the Georgia State Sanitarium, treated a series of twenty-seven cases in the insane at that asylum exclusively by diet. Considering the character of the cases with which he was dealing, his results, as well as those of Dr. D. G. Willets,[3] who for a time continued the work begun by Lorenz, were notably favorable.

When the various recent methods of treatment, each warmly advocated by its author, are critically reviewed in the light of the test made by Lorenz and by Willets, one can hardly fail to be impressed by the fact that the one thing they all appear to have in common is the so-called "nutritious" diet, and it is difficult to escape the conclusion that it is to this single common factor that the marked success that is usually claimed for the "treatment" should properly be assigned.

It is of much interest to note that fully fifty years ago Roussel,[4] on the basis of long experience and from a critical review of the literature of his day, came to precisely the same conclusion. This is so much to the point that it is quoted herewith:

Without dietetic measures *all remedies* fail. . . . When drugs and good food are simultaneously employed it is to the latter that the curative action belongs; the former exercises simply an adjuvant action and is without proved efficacy except against secondary changes or accidental complications.[5]

Hereafter the clinician who would attribute therapeutic value to any drug or other remedy in the treatment of pellagra should be prepared to show, what has not heretofore been done, that the curative effect claimed cannot be attributed to the diet. It is true that the claim is not infrequently made that the beneficial effects of the remedy advocated were obtained without any change in diet. When this claim is critically considered, however, it amounts usually simply to this, that the observer gave no instructions as to a change in the patient's diet, or assumes that such change as was made was too slight to merit consideration. It should not be overlooked that the symptoms of the disease (sore mouth, diarrhea) are very frequently such that the patient, entirely on his own initiative, may or does add or increase the proportion of the liquids (milk, eggs, broth) in his diet. And this may be done even before the physician is consulted.

Again, in order to substantiate the claims made for some particular remedy, it is sometimes asserted that the patient's diet had all along included an abundance of the animal proteins and legumes. Careful inquiry in a number of such instances has almost invariably shown that what is meant in such cases is that 'either the family table was known, or was assumed to be well supplied with these foods of which the patient was, perhaps quite naturally, assumed to have partaken abundantly. The important possibility that the patient, by reason of a personal idiosyncrasy or otherwise did not actually eat these foods is almost invariably overlooked. That these foods may, in some degree, enter into the pellagrogenous dietary calls, however, for no denial. The question always to be borne in mind is: Was it enough? The possibility, if not the probability, of a "twilight" zone within which a very slight change in any of the dietary components may cause an important shift of balance is not to be overlooked. In the present state of our knowledge, therefore, the question of a sufficient proportion cannot in all instances be answered on the simple statement of the case. That as a matter of fact the proportion of the foods in question in these, which may be called borderland cases, was not enough is very strongly suggested by the favorable result of the simple expedient of having the patient continue the diet on which he is supposed to have subsisted, seeing to it, however, that there is actually consumed an abundance of the animal foods and legumes. This and the unsatisfactory progress of those patients who for one reason or another fail or refuse to cooperate in taking the diet is decidedly illuminating.

Such observations as I have been able to make strongly suggest that real recovery from an uncomplicated attack may not take place until after a minimum of about three or four months of full feeding of fresh animal proteins and legumes. But this should not be taken to mean that thereafter recurrences are impossible. A "recurrence," so-called, may conceivably take place after the lapse of any interval if there is a return for a sufficiently long period to a pellagrogenous, that is, "faulty" diet. In pellagra, as in other conditions, the renewed operation of the essential causative factor may be expected to bring about a renewed manifestation of its effects.

---

1. Prof. Carl Voegtlin tells me that at about the same time, or even previous to this time, he had independently formed somewhat similar views, which he presented at the 1914 session of the American Medical Association (The Journal A. M. A., Sept. 26, 1914, p. 1094). The following quotations from this paper will give the student of the subject the essentials of Voegtlin's conception:

"From a survey of the clinical and pathologic aspects of pellagra, I have arrived at the conclusion that we are dealing with a chronic intoxication. While the agents at work in this intoxication are as yet unknown, I am inclined to believe that toxic substances exist in certain vegetable foods, not necessarily spoiled, which, if consumed by man over a long period of time, may produce an injurious effect on certain organs of the body. This hypothesis does not rule out the possibility that a dietary deficiency . . . [vitamin] . . . may play a rôle in the production and treatment of pellagra. Extensive feeding experiments which I have carried on during the last year with animals, such as mice, rats and a few monkeys, on an exclusive vegetable diet, have shown that these lower animals develop certain gastro-intestinal symptoms, and sometimes die if put on an exclusive diet of corn, carrots, sweet potatoes, oats, etc. Symptoms arise, often within three or four days, which point to the presence of an intoxication in these animals. Death resulted in some cases in a remarkably short time (three or four days). At necropsy constant lesions were found, such as hyperemia and hemorrhage in the gastro-intestinal canal. Sometimes the kidneys, lungs and other organs show a congestion and slightly hemorrhagic condition. . . ."

"It is probably more than a mere coincidence that the population of that part of the world in which pellagra is endemic lives on a mainly vegetable diet."

"The recent advances in the field of nutrition suggest new avenues of approach to the solution of this difficult problem. One will have to consider very seriously:

"1. A deficiency or absence of certain vitamins in the diet.
"2. The toxic effect of some substances, as aluminum, which occur in certain vegetable food."

"[The possible relation between aluminum and pellagra was also discussed in a recent monograph by Alessandrini and Scala (Contributo nuovo alla etiologia e pathogenesi della Pellagra, Roma, 1914) which I received at the time of proofreading. These investigators claim that colloidal silica contained in drinking water is one of the most important etiologic factors, inasmuch as they succeeded in producing lesions resembling pellagra in animals fed on water containing colloidal silica. Colloidal aluminum hydroxid or a mixture of colloidal silica and alumina produced the same results. In view of the fact, first discovered by us, that aluminum occurs in certain vegetable food in relatively large amounts, the work of the Italian authors furnishes additional evidence that aluminum occupies a prominent position in the etiology of pellagra.]"

"3. A deficiency of the diet in certain amino-acids."

2. Lorenz, W. F.: The Treatment of Pellagra, Pub. Health Rep., Sept. 11, 1914.
3. Willets, D. G.: The Treatment of Pellagra by Diet, South. Med. Jour., 1915, viii, 1044.
4. Roussel, Th. ophile: Traité de la pellagre et des pseudo-pellagres, Paris, 1866, p 529

5. The italics are Roussel's.

PREVENTION

In planning the test of the preventive value of diet, it was decided to take advantage of the universally recognized fact that "normally" pellagra tends to recur in the individual from year to year.

In order to obtain as significant and decisive results as possible, it was necessary to submit a large number of pellagrins to the test under known conditions. Fortunately, two orphanages were found in May, 1914, each having a high incidence of pellagra among its inmates. Later this preventive test was extended to include two groups of insane at the Georgia State Sanitarium.

In the study at the orphanages, Assistant Surgeon C. H. Waring was associated with me, and in that at the Georgia State Sanitarium, Assistant Epidemiologist D. G. Willets.

Orphanage Study.—The two orphanages at which the value of diet in the prevention of pellagra has been tested are located in Jackson, Miss. At both, cases of pellagra have been recognized for several years. During the spring and summer of 1914, up to September 15, a total of 209 cases of pellagra were observed in the children of these orphanages. Although a number of these at both institutions were known to be admission cases, others appeared to have developed first after considerable periods of residence, while a large proportion were in long time residents. The factor or factors causing pellagra and favoring its recurrence seemed, therefore, to be operative at both institutions.

At both places hygienic and sanitary conditions left much to be desired. Both were overcrowded. Each drew and has continued to draw its drinking water from the public supply. One has a water carriage sewerage system connected with that of the city; the other is provided only with unscreened privies. At the latter a great deal of soil pollution was noted.

Before beginning the test it was requested that no change be made in hygienic and sanitary conditions; this request, it is believed, has been fully complied with.

Since about the middle of September, 1914, the diet at both orphanages has in certain respects been supplemented by the Public Health Service. At both institutions a very decided increase was made in the proportion of the fresh animal and of the leguminous protein foods. The milk supply was greatly increased. The children between 6 and 12 years of age were provided with a cup of about 7 ounces of milk at least twice a day. Those under 6 had it three times a day. Until the spring of 1915, the milk used was all fresh sweet milk. In April of that year, buttermilk was added to the diet; this was served at first only on alternate days to those over 12 years of age; later it was served to all at the midday meal. Eggs, which had not previously entered into the regular diet of these children, were served those under 12 years of age at the morning meal. It had been the custom to serve fresh meat but once a week; this was increased to three or four times a week.

Beans and peas, which had been conspicuous in the diet only during the summer and fall, were made an important part of nearly every midday meal at all seasons. No canned foods other than tomatoes were allowed, in order to eliminate the possibly injurious action on the foods of the high temperatures to which they are necessarily subjected in the process.

The carbohydrate component of the institution diets was modified with the object of reducing the proportion of this element. In this connection it may be noted that though the corn component was much reduced, it was not wholly excluded. Corn bread was allowed all children once a week, and grits once or twice a week in addition to those over 12 years of age.

Of the 209 cases of pellagra observed at the two orphanages during the spring and summer of 1914, up to September 15, not less than 172 completed at least the anniversary date of their attack under observation. In only one of these 172 pellagrins, following the change of diet, was there recognized, during the year 1915, evidence justifying a diagnosis of a recurrence, although on the basis of Rice's[6] experience at an orphanage in Columbia, S. C., there might reasonably have been expected from 58 to 76 per cent., or from ninety-nine to 130 of them to recur. Furthermore, there was observed no new case in any of the nonpellagrin residents, 168 of whom were continuously under observation for at least one year. Recent admissions aside, during 1915 there has been no pellagra at one, and but a single case at the other of these institutions.

Asylum Study.—Through the courtesy and with the very helpful cooperation of the officers and staff of the Georgia State Sanitarium, two wards of pellagrins, one in the colored and the other in the white female service, were made available for the test.

Large numbers of cases of pellagra are observed annually at this institution, the largest in the South. A large proportion of these are admission cases, but cases of intramural origin are of frequent occurrence. This asylum must, therefore, be regarded as an endemic focus of the disease.

The wards were organized for this test late in the fall of 1914. In selecting the patients only one condition was observed, namely, that the patient should be of such type as would give reasonable degree of probability of remaining under observation for at least a year. In consequence, a considerable proportion were of a much deteriorated, untidy class.

The diet furnished the inmates of these two wards was, as at the orphanages, supplemented by the Public Health Service, and modified so as to increase decidedly the proportion of the animal and leguminous protein elements. A cup of about 7 ounces of sweet milk is furnished each patient for breakfast and one of buttermilk at both dinner and supper. Fully half a pound of fresh beef and 2 to 2½ ounces of dried field peas or dried beans enter the daily ration. In order to favor the consumption of milk, oatmeal has almost entirely replaced grits as the breakfast cereal. With a view of reducing the carbohydrate component, syrup has been entirely excluded. Corn products, although greatly reduced, have not been entirely eliminated. The menu that follows will serve to give a more detailed idea of the character of the diet furnished.

WEEKLY MENU

MONDAY

Breakfast.—Grits, sweet milk, sugar, broiled steak, hot rolls, biscuits, coffee.
Dinner.—Roast beef, gravy, peas, potatoes, rice, biscuits, buttermilk.
Supper.—Stewed apples, light bread, coffee, buttermilk, sugar.

---

6. Rice, quoted by Goldberger, Joseph; Waring, C. H., and Willets, D. C.: The Prevention of Pellagra, Pub. Health Rep., Oct. 22, 1915, p. 3117.

TUESDAY
Breakfast.—Oatmeal, sweet milk, sugar, Hamburger steak, biscuits, hot rolls, coffee.
Dinner.—Beef stew, potatoes, rice, bread, buttermilk.
Supper.—Baked beans, light bread, coffee, sugar, buttermilk.

WEDNESDAY
Breakfast.—Oatmeal, sweet milk, sugar, beef hash, hot rolls, biscuits, coffee.
Dinner.—Pea soup, corn bread, gravy, potatoes, rice, bread, buttermilk.
Supper.—Stewed prunes, light bread, coffee, sugar, buttermilk.

THURSDAY
Breakfast.—Oatmeal, sweet milk, sugar, fried steak, hot rolls, biscuits, coffee.
Dinner.—Beef stew, peas, potatoes, rice, bread, buttermilk.
Supper.—Baked beans, bread, coffee, sugar, buttermilk.

FRIDAY
Breakfast.—Oatmeal, sweet milk, sugar, broiled beef steak, hot rolls, biscuits, coffee.
Dinner.—Pea soup (purée), roast beef, potatoes, rice, bread, buttermilk.
Supper.—Light bread, coffee, sugar, buttermilk, apples, baked beans.

SATURDAY
Breakfast.—Oatmeal, sweet milk, sugar, Hamburger steak, hot rolls, biscuits, coffee.
Dinner.—Beef stew, potatoes, rice, bread, buttermilk.
Supper.—Bread, baked beans, buttermilk, coffee, sugar.

SUNDAY
Breakfast.—Oatmeal, sweet milk, sugar, mackerel, bread, coffee.
Dinner.—Loaf beef and gravy, peas, potatoes, rice, bread, buttermilk, pudding.
Supper.—Beef hash, bread, sugar, coffee, buttermilk.
NOTE.—Green vegetables in season at irregular intervals. Milk and eggs, as a special diet, are furnished those patients who may require them.

Aside from the modification in the diet and the increased watchfulness over the individual feeding, enjoined on the nurses and attendants, no change in the habitual routine of the corresponding services was made.

Of the pellagrins admitted to these wards at the time of their organization, or shortly thereafter — that is, up to Dec. 31, 1914 — seventy-two (thirty-six colored and thirty-six white) remained continuously under observation up to Oct. 1, 1915, or, at least, until after the anniversary date of their attack of 1914. Of the colored patients, eight have histories of at least two annual attacks; of the white patients, ten have histories of at least two attacks. Nevertheless not a single one of this group of seventy-two patients has presented recognizable evidence of a recurrence of pellagra, although of a group of thirty-two control pellagrins (seventeen colored and fifteen white) not receiving the modified diet, fifteen (nine colored, six white), or 47 per cent., have had recurrences during the corresponding period.

Significance.—Considering the foregoing results as a whole, bearing in mind that three different institutions are involved, each institution an endemic focus of the disease, and bearing in mind also that the number of individuals is fairly large, it would seem that the conclusion is justified that the pellagra recurrence may be prevented and, in view of the conditions of the experiment, that it may be prevented without the intervention of any other factor than diet. In this connection the question arises whether it is permissible to extend this conclusion to the primary attack, apart from its recurrence. The character of the answer to this question will depend on the view held as to the nature of the pellagra recurrence.

Among the epidemiologic features of pellagra, none is more striking than the tendency for the disease not only to develop in spring or early summer, but also to recur year after year at about the same season. Various explanations of this singular phenomenon have been advanced. According to Sambon,[7] "this peculiar periodicity of symptoms can be explained only by the agency of a parasitic organism presenting definite alternating periods of latency and activity." A somewhat similar conception appears to be held by the Thompson-McFadden Commission,[8] which distinguishes between conditions favorable for the development of the disease, in the first place, and those that permit its subsequent recurrence. Why these and many other observers should consider this periodicity of symptoms as explicable only by the agency of a parasitic organism or of a virus or a toxin presenting definite alternating periods of latency and activity is rather hard to understand when it is recalled that in endemic scurvy,[9] and particularly in endemic beriberi,[10] diseases of well known dietary origin, a strikingly similar periodicity is present. It would seem, therefore, entirely permissible to invoke as an explanation of the periodic recurrence in pellagra what undoubtedly is the explanation of the same phenomenon in these other diseases, namely, a modification or change in diet brought about by or incidental to the recurring seasons. Viewed in this light, the recurrence in pellagra may be considered as in beriberi, etiologically at least, as essentially identical with the initial attack; and therefore it would seem permissible to conclude that the means found effective in the prevention of recurrences will be found effective in the prevention of the initial attack.

NATURE OF THE DISEASE

In the course of the preliminary studies relating to the prevalence of pellagra at such institutions as prisons, asylums and orphanages, to which reference was made early in this paper, the association was found of a very high incidence of pellagra, restricted to certain groups, with a diet which differed from the diet of the exempt groups, so far as could be determined, only in that it included minimal quantities of the animal foods. It was inferred at that time that this association had etiologic significance. Advantage has been taken of an opportunity to put this inference to the test of experiment. The experiment was carried out in association with Assistant Surgeon G. A. Wheeler at the farm of the Mississippi State Penitentiary, about 8 miles east of Jackson, Miss.

At about the center of this farm of 3,200 acres, well isolated from the surrounding community, is the convict "camp." There is no history of the previous occurrence or presence of pellagra on this farm. During the period of the experiment there were quartered at the "camp" an average of between seventy and

---

7. Sambon, L. W.: Progress Report on the Investigation of Pellagra, Jour. Trop. Med. and Hyg., 1910.
8. Siler, J. F.; Garrison, P. E., and MacNeal, W. J.: The Relation of Methods of Disposal of Sewage to the Spread of Pellagra, Arch. Int. Med., October, 1914, p. 453; Further Studies of the Thompson-McFadden Pellagra Commission, THE JOURNAL A. M. A., Sept. 26, 1914, p. 1090; A Statistical Study of the Relation of Pellagra to Use of Certain Foods and to Location of Domicile in Six Selected Industrial Communities, Arch. Int. Med., September, 1914, p. 293.
9. Lind, James: A Treatise on the Scurvy, Ed. 3, London, 1772, pp. 33, 44, 130, 306.
10. Scheube, B.: The Diseases of Warm Countries, London, 1903.

eighty white male convicts, of whom about thirty were present throughout this time. Through the kind offices of Dr. E. H. Galloway, secretary of the Mississippi State Board of Health, the interest of Governor Earl Brewer was enlisted, who, on the offer of a pardon, obtained twelve volunteers for the test.

Experiment.—White adult males were selected because, judged by the incidence of the disease in the population at large, this age, sex and race group would seem to be the least susceptible to the disease.

The "pellagra squad," as it came to be called, was organized between Feb. 1 and Feb. 4, 1915, with twelve volunteers. July 1, 1915, one of the squad was released because of the development of a physical infirmity. This left eleven men in the squad, from 24 to 50 years of age, who remained in the test to its termination, Oct. 31, 1915. These men were quartered in a small, practically new, screened cottage, about 500 feet from the "cage" in which the other convicts were domiciled. Part of this cottage had previously been used, and continued to be used, throughout the period of the experiment as quarters for one of the officers of the "camp." From the time of its organization, the squad was segregated and under special guard.

From Feb. 4 to April 19, 1915, a period of two and one half months, these men were kept under observation without any change in the regular prison fare. As no evidence of pellagra during this preliminary observation period was detected, the diet of the squad was changed at noon, April 19, 1915. The ingredients of this diet were wheat flour (patent), corn meal, (corn) grits, corn starch, white polished rice, standard granulated sugar, cane syrup, sweet potatoes, pork fat (fried out of salt pork), cabbage, collards, turnip-greens and coffee. In the preparation of the biscuits and of the corn bread "Royal" baking powder was used.

The quantities of the different articles of cooked food actually consumed are illustrated by the following for the week ended Aug. 8, 1915: biscuits, 41.81 pounds; rice, 24.25 pounds; corn bread, 24.56 pounds; grits, 27.06 pounds; fried mush, 33.87 pounds; brown gravy, 37.81 pounds; sweet potatoes, 23.62 pounds; cabbage, 4.25 pounds; collards, 23.75 pounds; cane syrup, 5.94 pounds; sugar, 8.75 pounds, making a total of 255.67 pounds of food consumed during the week, or 3.32 pounds per man per day, having a value of 2,952 calories.

In this connection it may be pertinent to note that the corn meal and grits were of the best quality obtainable at the local market, and the same as that used at one of the orphanages at which the test, already discussed, of the value of diet in prevention, was made, and at which no pellagra occurred this year. Except for one meal in which 4 ounces of meat were included, the animal proteins and legumes were almost entirely excluded.

The character of the labor performed by these men during the week for which the statement of the quantity of food consumed has been given was as follows: whitewashing fences and buildings, two and one half days; sawing lumber (ram saw mill) two days; rest, two and one half days.

The volunteers kept about the same hours and did about the same kind of work as the other convicts. **The amount of labor performed by the volunteers, however, was distinctly less than that by the other convicts.**

The general sanitary environment was the same for volunteers and controls. With respect to personal cleanliness, cleanliness of quarters, and freedom from insects, particularly bedbugs, flies and mosquitoes, the volunteers were decidedly better off.

Results.—Of the eleven volunteers, not less than six developed symptoms, including a "typical" dermatitis, justifying a diagnosis of pellagra. Loss of weight and strength and mild nervous symptoms appeared early. The gastro-intestinal symptoms were slight. Definite cutaneous manifestations were not noted until September 12, or about five months after the beginning of the restricted diet. In all six cases the skin lesions were first noted on the scrotum. Later the eruption also appeared on the hands in two of the cases, and on the back of the neck in one. The scrotal lesion conformed to the type described and figured by Merk[11] and also by Stannus.[12]

Although the entire population of the "camp" was kept under observation, no one, not of the volunteer squad, presented evidence justifying even a suspicion of pellagra.

The diagnosis of pellagra was concurred in by Dr. E. H. Galloway, secretary of the Mississippi State Board of Health, and Dr. Nolan Stewart, formerly superintendent of the Mississippi Asylum for the Insane, at Jackson. In excluding the other known dermatoses, the expert knowledge and skill of Prof. Marcus Haase of the Medical College of the University of Tennessee, Memphis, Tenn., and of Prof. Martin F. Engman of the Washington University Medical School, St. Louis, were utilized in consultation.

Conclusions. — The conclusion drawn from this experiment is that pellagra has been brought about in at least six of the eleven volunteers as the result of the one-sided diet on which they subsisted. Taken in conjunction with the striking results of the test of the preventive value of diet, the further conclusion seems justified that pellagra is essentially of dietary origin.

In order to avoid misunderstanding, it may be well to point out that it does not necessarily follow that all one-sided, "unbalanced" or, as I prefer for the present to speak of them, "faulty" diets are capable of bringing about pellagra any more than they are of bringing about scurvy or beriberi.

A definite conclusion as to the intimate mechanism involved in bringing about or in preventing the disease by diet cannot, of course, be drawn from the available data. It would be premature to conclude that pellagra is necessarily due to a lack or deficiency of fresh animal or leguminous protein foods. Clearly, however, the dietary "fault" on which the production of pellagra essentially depends is capable of being corrected or prevented by including in the diet a suitable proportion of these foods. It would be equally premature, moreover, to assume that the pellagra-causing dietary "fault" is capable of correction in this way only. The possibility that there may be other foods capable of serving the same purpose is by no means to be overlooked. If Funk's[13] suggestion that pellagra is a vitamin deficiency, brought about by the consumption of overmilled corn, is proved to be correct, it may be, too, that the use of undermilled corn will of itself

---
11. Merk, Ludwig: Die Hauterscheinungen der Pellagra, Innsbruck, 1909, p. 24, Fig. 6.
12. Stannus, Hugh S.: Pellagra in Nyasaland, Tr. Soc. Trop. Med. and Hyg., 1913, vii, 32.
13. Funk, Casimir: Die Vitamine, Wiesbaden, 1914. Prophylaxie und Therapie der Pellagra ins Lichte der Vitaminlehre, München. med. Wchnschr., 1914, p. 698.

correct the "fault" in a diet in which this cereal is the staple. There is to be considered also Voegtlin's explanation of the beneficial effect of a liberal diet on the course of the disease. Voegtlin suggests that by substituting animal foodstuffs for part of the vegetable food the absolute amount of vegetable products consumed will be reduced considerably, and thus probably also reduce the possibility of an injurious action of the vegetable food on the body, particularly the irritant action on the gastro-intestinal canal. On the whole, however, the trend of available evidence strongly suggests that pellagra will prove to be a "deficiency" disease very closely related to beriberi.

For the practical purposes of preventive medicine, the point of chief, of fundamental, importance would seem to be the recognition of the fact that the pellagra-producing dietary "fault," whatever its intimate nature or however brought about, is capable of correction or prevention, as the results of the studies summarized above clearly indicate, by including in the diet suitable proportions of the fresh animal and leguminous protein foods.[14]

SUMMARY

1. Diet is the common factor in the various methods of treatment recently advocated. The marked success claimed for each of these methods must logically be attributed to the factor (diet) which they have in common.

2. The value of diet in the prevention of pellagra has been tested at two orphanages and at an asylum for the insane, endemic foci of the disease. Marked increases in the fresh animal and leguminous protein elements of the institution diets were made.

Of 209 cases of pellagra observed at the two orphanages during the spring and summer of 1914, not less than 172 completed at least the anniversary date of their attack under observation. In only one of these 172 pellagrins, following the change in diet, was there recognized evidence of a recurrence, although on the basis of experience elsewhere, from ninety-nine to 130 might reasonably have been expected. Nor was any new case observed among the nonpellagrin residents, 168 of whom completed not less than one year under observation.

Of the group of pellagrins on the modified diet at the insane asylum, seventy-two remained continuously under observation up to Oct. 1, 1915, or at least until after the anniversary date of their attack of 1914. Not one of this group has presented recognizable evidence of a recurrence, although, of a group of thirty-two controls, fifteen have had recurrences. Pellagra may, therefore, be prevented by an appropriate diet without any alteration in the environment, hygienic or sanitary, including the water supply.

3. At an isolated convict camp, previously free from pellagra, with an average population of from seventy to eighty white males, eleven volunteers were segregated and, after a preliminary observation period of two and one half months, placed on an abundant but one-sided, chiefly carbohydrate (wheat, corn, rice) diet, from which fresh animal proteins and legumes were excluded. At least six of these volunteers developed pellagra. This result would appear to have been brought about by the diet on which they subsisted.

4. A definite conclusion as to the intimate mechanism involved in bringing about or in preventing the disease by diet cannot be drawn from the available data.

5. For the practical purposes of preventive medicine, it would seem to be of fundamental importance to recognize that the pellagra-producing dietary "fault," whatever its intimate nature or however brought about, is capable of correction or prevention by including in the diet suitable proportions of the fresh animal and leguminous protein foods.

---

14. In addition to the references already given, the following will be found of interest:
Goldberger, Joseph: The Etiology of Pellagra: the Significance of Certain Epidemiological Observations with Respect Thereto, Pub. Health Rep., Washington, June 26, 1914, p. 1683; The Cause and Prevention of Pellagra, ibid., Sept. 11, 1914; Beans for Prevention of Pellagra, THE JOURNAL A. M. A., Oct. 10, 1914, p. 1314.
Goldberger, Joseph; Waring, C. H., and Willets, D. G.: The Treatment and Prevention of Pellagra, Pub. Health Rep., Oct. 23, 1914, p. 126; Reprint 228 from Pub. Health Rep.; id. revised Jan. 15, 1915.
Goldberger, Joseph, and Wheeler, G. A.: Experimental Pellagra in the Human Subject Brought About by a Restricted Diet, Pub. Health Rep., Nov. 12, 1915, p. 3336.
Meyers, C. N., and Voegtlin, Carl: Soluble Aluminum Compounds: Their Occurrence in Certain Vegetable Products, Pub. Health Rep., June 19, 1914, p. 1625.

PUBLIC HEALTH IN AMERICA

An Arno Press Collection

Ackerknecht, Erwin H[einz]. **Malaria In the Upper Mississippi Valley: 1760-1900.** 1945

Bowditch, Henry I[ngersoll]. **Consumption In New England Or, Locality One of Its Chief Causes** and **Is Consumption Contagious, Or Communicated By One Person to Another In Any Manner?** 1862/1864. Two Vols. in One.

Buck, Albert H[enry] (Editor). **A Treatise On Hygiene and Public Health.** 1879. Two Vols.

Boston Medical Commission. **The Sanitary Condition of Boston:** The Report of a Medical Commission. 1875

Budd, William. **Typhoid Fever:** Its Nature, Mode of Spreading, and Prevention. 1931

Chapin, Charles V[alue]. **A Report On State Public Health Work,** Based On a Survey of State Boards of Health: Made Under the Direction of the Council on Health and Public Instruction of the American Medical Association. [1915]

Davis, Michael M[arks], Jr. and Andrew R[obert] Warner. **Dispensaries:** Their Management and Development. 1918

Dublin, Louis I[srael] and Alfred J. Lotka. **The Money Value of a Man.** 1930

Dunglison, Robley. **Human Health.** 1844

Emerson, Haven. **Local Health Units for the Nation.** 1945

Emerson, Haven. **A Monograph On the Epidemic of Poliomyelitis (Infantile Paralysis) In New York City In 1916.** 1917

Fish, Hamilton. **Report of the Select Committee of the Senate of the United States On the Sickness and Mortality On Board Emigrant Ships.** 1854

Frost, Wade Hampton. **The Papers of Wade Hampton Frost, M.D.:** A Contribution to Epidemiological Method. 1941

Gardner, Mary Sewall. **Public Health Nursing.** 1916

Greenwood, Major. **Epidemics and Crowd Diseases:**
An Introduction to the Study of Epidemiology. 1935

Greenwood, Major. **Medical Statistics From Graunt to Farr.**
1948

Hartley, Robert M. **An Historical, Scientific and Practical Essay On Milk, As an Article of Human Sustenance:** With a Consideration of the Effects Consequent Upon the Unnatural Methods of Producing It for the Supply of Large Cities. 1842

Hill, Hibbert Winslow. **The New Public Health.** 1916

Knopf, S. Adolphus. **Tuberculosis As a Disease of the Masses & How To Combat It.** 1908

MacNutt, J[oseph] Scott. **A Manual for Health Officers.** 1915

Richards, Ellen H. [Swallow]. **Euthenics:** The Science of Controllable Environment. 1910

Richardson, Joseph G[ibbons]. **Long Life and How To Reach It.** 1886

Rumsey, Henry Wyldbore. **Essays On State Medicine.** 1856

Shryock, Richard Harrison. **National Tuberculosis Association 1904-1954:** A Study of the Voluntary Health Movement In the United States. 1957

Simon, John. **Filth-Diseases and Their Prevention.** 1876

Sternberg, George M[iller]. **Sanitary Lessons of the War and Other Papers.** 1912

Straus, Lina Gutherz. **Disease In Milk:** The Remedy Pasteurization. The Life Work of Nathan Straus. 1917

Wanklyn, J[ames] Alfred and Ernest Theophron Chapman. **Water Analysis:** A Practical Treatise on the Examination of Potable Water. 1884

Whipple, George C. **State Sanitation:** A Review of the Work of the Massachusetts State Board of Health. 1917. Two Vols. in One.

Selections From Public Health Reports and Papers Presented at the Meetings of the American Public Health Association (1873-1883). 1977

Selections From Public Health Reports and Papers Presented at the Meetings of the American Public Health Association (1884-1907). 1977

Animalcular and Cryptogamic Theories On the Origins of Fevers. 1977

The Carrier State. 1977

Clean Water and the Health of the Cities. 1977

The First American Medical Association Reports On Public Hygiene In American Cities. 1977

Selections from the Health-Education Series. 1977

Health In the Southern United States. 1977

Health In the Twentieth Century. 1977

The Health of Women and Children. 1977

Minutes and Proceedings from the First, Second, Third and Fourth National Quarantine and Sanitary Conventions. 1977. Four Vols. in Two.

Selections from the Journal of the Massachusetts Association of Boards of Health (1891-1904). 1977

Sewering the Cities. 1977

Smallpox In Colonial America. 1977

Yellow Fever Studies. 1977